IN
SICKNESS

A Memoir

BARRETT ROLLINS

Post Hill
PRESS

Post Hill Press
New York • Nashville
posthillpress.com

Published in the United States of America
1 2 3 4 5 6 7 8 9 10

Content warning:
This book contains a depiction
of suicidal ideation.

I take the to my weddyd wyf, to have and to hold fro thys day forwarde, for better for wors, for richer for porer, in sikenesse and in helthe, tyl deth us departe, yf holy Chyrche wyl it ordeyne; and thereto I plyght the my trouthe.

—**Saint Osmund**, Bishop of Salisbury,
Use of Sarum, 1085

ONE

Friday. At last.

My reward for surviving another week at work was "Date Night"—that's what Jane called our ritual of going out for dinner every Friday. Even after thirty years of marriage, we couldn't wait to sit together and rehash the week's events at one of the handful of Boston restaurants she could tolerate. But what Jane loved more than dinner was what came next. As soon as we were home, she'd burst through the front door and shout, "Guess what time it is.... It's bedtime!"

She'd undress, crawl under the covers, turn on the television, and remain horizontal until the exigencies of Monday morning forced her back on her feet. I've never known anyone who loved sleep as much as Jane did. I was her enabler, of course, bringing her meals in bed and nudging her awake at intervals to make sure she'd eat something. I liked being her servant, seeing how happy I could make her.

For tonight's Date Night, I'd made reservations at Casa Romero, our favorite Mexican restaurant. Having checked that box, I felt like my week was over. I was ready to leave. Unfortunately, it was only noon, so I still had lunch and a whole afternoon of meetings to get through.

Jane and I worked at the same place—we were doctors at Dana-Farber Cancer Institute, Harvard's cancer hospital—and we'd arranged our schedules so that we could have lunch together every day, a tradition that was now in its twentieth year. Although our lunches had begun as private affairs, they'd grown to include several of our colleagues.

It was really Jane who attracted the rotating cast of a dozen or so coworkers who joined us at various times. Her conversation—liberally seasoned with insightful and often hilarious commentary—was infinitely appealing, as was her biting wit. But Jane also set strict rules: you could talk about politics or Dana-Farber chitchat, but you could not talk about your own work. Her prohibition was rooted in a visceral aversion to hearing about the kind of laboratory research that most of us did. While her prejudice could have been alienating, it instead had a salutary effect—the conversation was inclusive, wide-ranging, and never dull.

It made for a raucous time. At first, the senior faculty, who were not part of our group, worried that the cadre of Young Turks laughing conspiratorially around a crowded lunch table was fomenting revolution. Our department chair would sniff derisively, but nervously, about the goings-on at "Jane's High Table." He had no cause for alarm—we were mostly just gossiping—but we loved the idea that we were striking fear into the hearts of our elders. Twenty years on, we had become the elders, but the lunchtime gatherings were still alive and well.

So, at noon on that sunny September Friday in 2012, I walked out of my office to meet my wife for lunch.

Dana-Farber Cancer Institute, or "the Farber" as it's called by those in the know, is one of those hospitals whose physical plant evolved haphazardly as money was found to put up new buildings. Its hodgepodge of structures is connected by bridges and hallways in such a way that the third floor of each building forms the Institute's main thoroughfare. As usual, I met Jane where my building's third-floor hallway joined hers, and we walked together down the marble promenade of the Farber's newest addition toward the Dining Pavilion—what lesser hospitals might call a cafeteria.

Fridays usually put Jane in a good mood but, as we walked together, I could see that something was wrong. Jane was very tall and thin, and she walked with a lanky person's loping stride. She'd slowed a bit now that she was sixty, but today she was straggling. Even at my customary "Jane-adjusted shuffle"—the unhurried cadence I'd adopted to match hers—I was outpacing her.

I slowed down and asked over my shoulder, "Are you okay, hon?"

"Yeah, yeah," she replied without looking at me, "no problem."

But there was a problem. Her face was ashen and her lips were tinged blue. As we turned the corner in front of the Dining Pavilion, Jane abruptly sat on a low bench that I had always thought was too small to be anything other than ornamental. I leaned over to get a better look at her. She was breathing rapidly and had the sort of bug-eyed, frightened look you see on the faces of asthmatics who are terrified by their inability to breathe.

"Hon, you look like you're having some serious trouble," I said.

No reply. Just more shallow panting.

I had never seen Jane like this. I had no idea what was bothering her, but her distress was palpable.

"Listen," I said, "I don't know what's going on, but I think we should get you to the ER."

The Farber doesn't have its own emergency room but its warren of third-floor hallways and bridges were connected to Brigham and Women's, the large general hospital next door. We could take that route to the Brigham's ER.

Jane looked up at me and nodded. That was a shock. In all our years together, Jane never, ever wanted to see a doctor or have medical care for anything. The fact that she wasn't arguing with me was unnerving.

There was no way Jane could walk to the Brigham so I looked around for a wheelchair. There were none to be seen.

"Some hospital," I muttered to myself.

The Farber's Dining Pavilion is in the same building as its outpatient clinics. The bench Jane was sitting on was next to the elevators that service those clinics, so I took her hands in mine, looked her in the eyes, and—trying not to betray my fear—told her that I was going to get a wheelchair and that I'd be right back.

I hurried to one of the elevators and jumped in just as the doors closed. I pushed the button for the seventh floor, the nearest clinic, and held my breath. When the doors opened, I ran out. My look of wild-eyed panic must have made the nurses think I was deranged. I scanned the clinic's waiting area but, again, no wheelchair.

Now I was frantic about having left Jane alone. I needed to get back to her. Instead of waiting for an elevator, I found a stairwell and flew down four flights, telling myself that I'd figure out some way to get her to the ER.

When I reached the third floor, I sped down the same marble hallway where Jane and I had been walking just minutes earlier. Rounding the corner in front of the Dining Pavilion, I was met by a horrific sight. Jane was sprawled on the bench where I'd left her. It was far too short for her height, so her head and legs draped awkwardly over its ends. Her eyes were closed and she was moaning rhythmically and loudly. A small crowd had gathered but no one was doing anything. They all knew Jane—everybody at the Farber knew Jane—but they'd been turned to stone by the transformation of their colleague and friend into a distressed patient.

I didn't know what to do either. This semi-conscious woman moaning loudly on the bench wasn't just anyone. This was Jane, my partner of thirty years. What was happening? Was she dying? She sure looked like she was dying. I desperately wanted to help her, but I couldn't suppress my fear and confusion long enough to think straight. All of the usual tricks we doctors use to create a self-protective distance between an acutely suffering patient and our own psyches—a space that allows us to make an objective, rational plan to help—weren't working. They couldn't work. This was Jane.

4

I knelt next to her and cradled her head. Her eyes stayed closed, and she just kept moaning. The sound was otherworldly and terrifying.

"We need to call a code," someone said softly in my ear.

He wanted to summon the emergency rescue team that responds to cardiac arrests. My god, these people think she's dying too. I wanted to do something useful but all I could think of was to stroke her forehead.

A moment later, I heard the announcement over the public address system: "Adult Medical Response Team to the Dining Pavilion." *What an odd place for a code*, I thought, until I realized who it was for.

After what felt like an hour but was only a few minutes, the code team arrived with their crash cart—a cabinet on wheels containing emergency medications and equipment. Someone on the team gently nudged me out of the way as he put an oxygen mask on Jane. Even through the mask, I could hear her moan with each breath. Two members of the team laid her flat on the ground and a third put in an intravenous line. All my usual instincts in this setting—to help insert another IV, to start the electrocardiogram, to prepare the medications—felt wrong. Those actions were meant to help other people, not my wife. I stood helplessly to one side.

Code teams are led by senior physicians who bark orders, military style, to the troops. The leader that day was Lisa, someone Jane and I had known for decades. Lisa was authoritative and radiated competence but, every few minutes, she would look at me, her face betraying a mixture of concern, bewilderment, and terror. I could only muster a blank stare in return.

At some point during the resuscitation efforts, a small trickle of blood appeared on the right side of Jane's neck just under her shirt collar. It looked like it was coming from her chest. Lisa pointed to it and looked at me with a raised eyebrow that clearly said, "What the hell is that?" I gave a slight shrug and a shake of my head as if to reply, "I have no idea."

Did I know where the blood was coming from? Maybe...no...I'll think about that later.

After ten minutes of frenzied activity, Jane was no better. She had lost consciousness—her moaning had stopped—and her blood pressure was low. She was getting fluids through her IV and oxygen through her mask, but she would need to be moved to the ER for more intensive treatment. For liability and, I suppose, good medical reasons, Dana-Farber's policy was not to transport unstable patients through the hallways to the Brigham. Instead, a Boston city ambulance would have to convey her across the two hundred yards that separated the Farber from the Brigham.

Someone had already called the ambulance, and it soon arrived with lights flashing and sirens wailing. A minute later, two EMTs appeared and muscled aside the code team. With reassuring efficiency, they hoisted my unconscious wife onto a gurney and sped her into a waiting elevator. At street level, they loaded her into the ambulance and took off for the emergency room.

The EMTs said they wanted to transport Jane without me. I was too flummoxed to argue, but as soon as they drove away, I started worrying that she might die in the ambulance. Or what if she didn't die? What if she woke up? She'd be terrified and I wouldn't be there to comfort her. Those thoughts kept pinging around in my head as I walked alone through the third-floor hallways and bridges to the Brigham ER.

A lot of time had passed since I'd taken care of patients in the Brigham ER—I was now a researcher and administrator—and the hospital had undergone major renovations since then. So, as I emerged from the bridge connecting Dana-Farber to the Brigham, I realized that I had no idea where the ER was. It certainly wasn't where it used to be. I was lost.

Someone must have taken pity on me and pointed me in the right direction because my next memory places me at a nursing station in the ER, just outside the treatment room where the EMTs had taken Jane. Looking through the open door, I could see her lying on a bed. The ER staff must have thought that she was in pretty bad shape because, in the short time it had taken me to walk over, they had inserted a breathing tube into her trachea and put her on a mechanical ventilator.

My wife was intubated and on a "vent." This was inconceivable. I tried not to think about what would happen if she were to die; the implications were too horrible. I needed to get through this acute crisis first. Then I'd be able to think about the future. For now, I told myself, just put one foot in front of the other.

From my vantage point outside the treatment room, I had clocked the breathing tube and ventilator right away. What took a little longer to register was the thing on Jane's chest. The ER workers had removed Jane's clothes and partially covered her with a hospital gown, one of those "johnnies" that opens in the back. They were bustling around her, putting in more IV lines and hooking her up to a heart monitor. In their haste, they had left Jane's chest partially uncovered.

Even at a distance of fifty feet, I could see a large, irregular black object on the right side of her chest. It was about the size of a football. Angrily, I wondered if some callous ER worker had left a piece of equipment there, using Jane's body as a table.

No, that wasn't it. The thing seemed to be attached to her, growing right out of her chest where her breast should have been.

What the fuck is that?

With a sickening rush, I got it. It was a breast cancer—and it was enormous, a massive tumor that had turned black because it was infected and rotting. *Oh, my god, this thing is out of control and it's killing Jane.*

My head reeling, I started walking toward Jane's treatment room when one of the ER doctors stopped me.

"Are you the husband?"

I swiveled to face him.

"Yes," I replied.

"What's the story?"

"Well," I said, "she collapsed while we were walking to lunch. She looked like she was having serious trouble breathing."

"I know about that," he said dismissively. "We think she probably had a large pulmonary embolus," a blood clot lodged in the vessels of the lung. "I'm asking about the mass on her chest. What's her cancer history?"

Did I know anything about Jane's cancer history? Maybe...not really...can't talk about it.... I froze for a few seconds, a deer in the headlights.

"Sorry, I really don't know," I finally murmured.

I felt humiliated and angry that an old, ill-considered promise to Jane made it look as though I, her husband, knew nothing about the hideous cancer that was threatening her life.

I watched the ER doctor's face as he processed my response. It took him a few seconds to figure out what to say next.

"Okay. Well, like I said, she probably had a PE. We're guessing that it's pretty massive because her numbers are terrible. Her pO_2 is low, even on one hundred percent oxygen through the ventilator, and her pH is only six point eight."

He was giving me Jane's blood test results doctor-to-doctor, figuring that I would know what they meant. I'm sure that slipping into "professional communication mode" was a way for him to avoid having to think about the bizarre situation he had stumbled upon. But he was right: I did understand the numbers. Jane was having an even harder time breathing than anyone had realized, and her body's metabolism was severely out of whack. Back when I was a clinician,

I had taken care of a few patients with these kinds of numbers. They were all intubated in the intensive care unit, and they all died.

"We're going to take her to radiology," he continued, "for a CT-angio." They were planning a CT scan plus an angiogram to look for the pulmonary embolus. "If there's a clot, we'll try to break it up with TPA"—a drug that dissolves clots, it would be the fastest way to try to restore blood flow to Jane's lungs—"but if that doesn't work, we'll have to take her to emergency surgery to remove the clot."

Emergency surgery? Things were spinning out of control. The rational part of my brain understood perfectly well what I was being told. Jane had become a big, complicated medical case that required an all-hands-on-deck response. We used to call this a "flail," and there was no doubt that taking an unstable, intubated patient to radiology to perform a CT-angio would be a huge flail. And I was grateful that the team was willing to make the effort. But this was Jane. The ER doctor had the luxury of putting some of that handy psychic distance between himself and the patient. I didn't. I was still stunned and felt like I was being carried downstream by a swift current that I was too weak to fight.

TWO

I stood uneasily next to Jane's bed in the treatment room, holding on to the siderail with one hand to steady myself while I waited for the transport team to fetch her. Every few minutes, I stole a glance at her chest. Her johnnie now covered her properly, but its awkward draping hinted at the huge lump underneath. I didn't think I could pull it aside with all these ER workers around. That would be too personal, too private. And, honestly, I was afraid to look at the tumor.

Doing nothing but waiting felt demoralizing—it was too passive. I needed to do *something*, to take some kind of concrete action. So, after the team rolled Jane into the hallway to take her to radiology, I walked to the nursing station and called Casa Romero to cancel our dinner reservations. A truly pathetic gesture, but it's all I had.

Now at loose ends, I wandered back into the empty treatment room. The floor was littered with discarded gloves, sterile wrappers for IV needles, crumpled sheets, and blood—the typical detritus of a resuscitation effort. I had seen these messes a hundred times before but this one looked different. I stood in the center of the room, lost in thought.

I suddenly became aware that the ER doctor was next to me. How long had he been standing there?

"She's going to be in radiology for a while," he said. "Why don't you give me your cell number? Go relax somewhere. We'll call you as soon as she's back."

Relax? Was he serious?

10

Before I could offer a snarky reply, I looked up and saw someone I knew walking through the ER. Ralph was a guy I had trained with more than thirty years earlier. Sadly, we'd lost touch—it had been ages since I had seen him—but I still had fond memories of the friendship we had formed during the bootcamp-like years of our internship and residency. Ralph had been a true humanist. He always had exactly the right take on whatever medical situation he and his patients were dealing with, no matter how horrible or frightening. Apparently, he was now on staff at the Brigham. Could anyone else have been a more welcome sight?

Well, yes. Just then, the one other person who was at least as welcome as Ralph saw me and waved. Rob ran the bone marrow transplant service at the Farber and the Brigham, which included some of the sickest patients you could imagine. Somehow, he, too, had maintained his humanity in the face of all that suffering. It helped that he was the funniest person I'd ever met and that we had long ago bonded over our love of obscure old movies.

Ralph had just finished evaluating a patient for possible admission to the hospital; Rob was wrapping up a visit with one of his transplant patients. They were both surprised to see me in the ER.

I tried to tell them why I was there, what was happening with Jane. But putting the day's events into words was forcing me to confront all the horror, sadness, and fear that I had been working so hard to suppress. As I worked to fashion a coherent story, each twist and turn served up a new reminder that Jane was in desperate straits and was likely to die, and that I might have to find a way to go on without her. Tears welled, and I kept having to interrupt the story to gather myself.

Ralph and Rob took control. They frog-marched me to the cafeteria—no "Dining Pavilion" at the lower-rent Brigham—where they bought me a cup of coffee. Without announcing their intentions explicitly, the two of them stayed with me for the next few hours. Dinnertime came and went. They should have left long ago for their own Date Nights, but instead they stuck out the wait with me. This was an extraordinary act of kindness and one that I've often revisited.

Eventually, I got the call that the CT-angiogram was done and Jane was back in the ER. Good. That meant she was still alive. I thanked Ralph and Rob profusely. They hugged me and went back to their lives. I turned in the opposite direction and headed for the ER.

As I entered the ER, I was met by a new doctor, someone with evident seniority, who introduced himself and asked me to accompany him. He led me through a maze of hallways, finally ushering me into a small room that was unfurnished except for a chair and a desk with an oversized computer screen. Seated there was the angiographer, the person who had performed Jane's procedure. He brought up the images of the CT-angiogram.

"The clot was huge," he said, looking at the screen. "It was a saddle embolus." I remembered from my training that this was the term for an enormous blood clot that, as if perched on a riding saddle, straddles the two main vessels that bring blood to the lungs. No wonder she was in such bad shape. As I absorbed the news, I tried, as I had been doing all day, not to display emotion. It seemed the safest strategy for now—I'd deal with my feelings later. I said nothing and waited for the angiographer to continue.

"Fortunately," he said, "we were able to bust up the clot at least partially with TPA. She's getting much better pulmonary arterial flow and her blood pressure is coming up, but we'll have to monitor her closely over the next few days to see whether the clot continues to dissolve while we give her more intravenous TPA. If it doesn't, we'll have to go back and try again, or perhaps we'll have to operate."

Okay, this was the first good news I'd heard, although Jane was clearly not out of the woods.

"Now," he said with a hint of hesitation, "let's talk about a few other things the CT scan showed." He stole a sideways glance at me, then looked at his colleague.

"Umm, first," he continued, addressing the screen, "the right breast is completely replaced by a fifteen-by-seven-centimeter mass that is anchored to the chest wall."

Fifteen by seven centimeters...how big is that? Oh, right, that's the football-sized thing I saw on her chest.

"Then, um, there are several large, abnormal lymph nodes in her mediastinum."

This was getting worse. He was saying that Jane's cancer had spread to lymph nodes in the center of her chest.

Now, like the ER doctor who had told me about Jane's blood test results, the angiographer soothed himself by slipping into hyper-professional technospeak.

"There's extensive right axillary lymphadenopathy suggestive of metastasis. The right lung shows metastatic nodules as well as septal thickening consistent with lymphangitic carcinomatosis. There's extensive pleural thickening on both sides likely due to metasta-ses. The liver shows several metastatic nodules, and I'm concerned about some of these lesions in the ribs and sternum, which are prob-ably metastases too."

Metastases, metastases, metastases—each time he said the word it was like a hammer blow. I had used that same word with my patients to describe how their cancers had invaded their organs, but now we were talking about Jane.

The angiographer paused, suddenly self-conscious.

I stared at the screen. I wanted to look away but I couldn't think of where. Right in front of me was a portrait of Jane's death. In high definition, it showed incurable, terminal cancer. Even if she survived her pulmonary embolus, the cancer would kill her soon enough. I couldn't believe how quickly and horribly our lives had changed. I felt as though the person I used to be had abruptly ceased to exist. I was living someone else's life.

I decided that the only way I could handle these shocks was to remain stoic, show no emotion, and try to interact with these doctors using my professional persona. So, I nodded my head, thanked the angiographer, and shook his hand.

As I left the office, the ER doctor was right next to me.

"Your wife needs to be transferred to the intensive care unit," he said. "The ICU team is already here to evaluate her."

As we reentered the ER, another physician approached me. He looked young enough to be in training, probably a resident.

"We're ready to take your wife up to the ICU. Want to follow us?"

I took up my post next to Jane's hospital bed and watched as a respiratory therapist disconnected the tube in Jane's mouth from the ventilator that had been breathing for her. In its place he attached a large, black rubber bag and began squeezing it rhythmically. Now he was breathing for her. Her intravenous medications were transferred from tall, freestanding poles to shorter ones on the corners of the bed. A nurse handed me a plastic bag containing Jane's torn and bloody clothes.

Then we were off. We moved as a unit: Jane on her bed, the resident, the respiratory therapist, a nurse, and me, carrying Jane's belongings, bringing up the rear. I was surprised, considering Jane's profoundly unstable condition, how slowly and deliberately we moved, no one saying a word. Like me, the team members seemed to be dealing with this ghastly situation by maintaining their professional demeanor. We wound our way through eerily empty hallways and crammed ourselves into a freight elevator.

We reached the third floor of the Brigham's clinical tower. The resident walked ahead and tapped a metal plate in the wall. With a low *whoosh*, the large double doors to the ICU parted. These were the same doors I used to open twenty-five years ago when I would check on my patients in the ICU. In those days, moving a cancer patient to intensive care was an act of desperation, something nervous oncologists did when their acutely ill patients were near death. Jane had spent her professional life arguing against that kind of uncomfortable, high-tech, end-of-life maneuver. Now she was one of those patients.

The team carefully maneuvered Jane's bed through a narrow hallway and into the room she'd been assigned. I followed them, awash in the cacophony of beeping heart monitors and IV alarms, the ambient music of an intensive care unit.

As the nurses transferred Jane into her bed and reconnected her to a mechanical ventilator, Tony, the senior physician in charge of the ICU, tapped me on the shoulder and motioned for me to follow him. I remembered him from his days as a Brigham resident when I used to teach at the hospital. We sat down in a small office next to the ICU.

"I know this looks bad," he said, "but they did a good job dissolving the clot and her oxygen levels are improving. No question, though, she still has serious problems with her heart and lungs, and we'll have to work on that. If you need anything at all, just have the nurses call me. I'll be here all night." Tony radiated reassurance.

"Wait," I said. "There is one more thing."

Now that Jane had survived her embolus, I had a new worry. She had clearly been keeping her breast cancer a secret—she'd hidden it from me and I was sure that she was hiding it from everyone else too. I had to assume that, if she were conscious, she would want to continue to control the flow of information.

But how could I keep the news about her breast cancer from spreading? How could I prevent the gossip from metastasizing? I knew that, ultimately, any attempt to suppress the facts would be futile—the mass would be obvious to her caregivers, and the CT scan had documented the extent of her cancer—but, for now, Jane was unconscious and I was her proxy.

"This will sound a little odd," I finally said, "but Jane would not want her colleagues to know about her breast cancer. At least not yet. As long as it doesn't compromise her care, could I ask you not to talk to anyone at the Farber about it? Would that be possible?"

Tony looked nonplussed.

"Of course," he said, snapping back into focus. "I won't speak to anyone outside of the ICU about Jane unless it's absolutely necessary."

Tony avoided looking at me as I thanked him and walked out of his office.

I went back to Jane's room. The staff had finished hooking her up to her life-support systems. She looked surprisingly small behind her breathing apparatus and IV tubing. Now her own heart monitor was beeping steadily. I glanced around the room and noticed that one of Jane's IV bags contained a thick, opaque white liquid that looked like a milkshake. I asked a nurse what it was, and he told me it was Propofol, a short-acting sedative used to calm patients who are on mechanical ventilation.

Propofol! That was the drug that killed Michael Jackson! I only knew this because of Jane. She was fascinated by scandalous, high-profile murders involving figures like OJ, the Menendez brothers, and Michael Jackson. Sensational TV programs about these cases riveted her. All I wanted at that moment was to be able to tell Jane that she was getting the Michael Jackson drug. I could almost hear the laugh I knew so well. But, of course, there was no laugh. Jane was unconscious and mortally ill. There was no reaching her.

I decided to make myself feel better by taking action again. Yes, Jane wanted to maintain her privacy, but she had advanced, life-threatening cancer. She needed an oncologist. Even if she were to wake up and decide that she didn't want any treatment for her cancer, the ICU team would still need an oncologist to help them manage her care. So, my task was to identify someone with enough expertise to handle Jane's difficult case but with enough discretion to respect her privacy.

The only person who fit the bill was Eric, the director of Dana-Farber's breast cancer center. Jane and I had known him for decades and had watched proudly as he built his center into one of the top programs in the world. Jane had even worked with him on research projects. I was aware that they'd had scientific disagreements over the years but no outright battles. Besides, Eric was the best breast cancer doctor in Boston and I knew he could keep a secret. A hemophiliac, Eric had acquired HIV from transfused blood and had kept careful watch over how this information was shared. He would understand Jane's need for privacy.

It was now about nine thirty on a Friday night, but I emailed Eric anyway, asking if I could speak to him as soon as possible, and gave him my cell number. My phone rang almost immediately—Eric was at a meeting in San Francisco, where it was dinner time. I told him to hold on for a minute while I went into the hall outside the ICU.

"Listen," I said, "the situation is very complicated. Jane had a massive pulmonary embolus this afternoon; she's intubated in the ICU. The reason I emailed you is that she also has widely metastatic breast cancer. She needs an oncologist."

I choked back a sob while I waited for Eric to respond.

"This is horrible. It's just horrible," he said. "How do you know she has breast cancer?"

I described the mass and the CT scan that had shown how widely the disease had spread.

"Okay, okay. Jesus. I'll be back tomorrow night and I'll come right from the airport to see her. Meanwhile, if there's an emergency, Ian is covering for me and you can call him." I had no intention of calling Ian or anyone else. "How are you doing?"

I said I was doing well enough, which was, of course, a lie. I also told Eric that Jane was getting superb care and that there was no rush to make decisions about treating her cancer, so he could come by Sunday or even Monday after he was back from California. He laughed and said he'd see me tomorrow night.

Telling Eric about Jane's breast cancer felt like a betrayal. I knew that she was as sick as anyone could possibly be and that the only way to save her life was to have a team of smart doctors taking care

17

of her, a team that included an oncologist. I knew I had done the right thing, but I still felt like I had let Jane down by revealing her secret to Eric.

I made my way back to Jane's room and stood once again at her bedside. The nurses and technicians had finished their chores and had left to tend to their other patients. I was alone with Jane for the first time since she'd collapsed on our way to lunch. I'd avoided looking directly at her face all day, afraid that would narrow the emotional distance I'd created to keep me on my feet. It might personalize the catastrophe to a degree I was unprepared for.

I was right. I looked hard at Jane, really looked at her, and all the terror and grief I'd been holding at bay was released. My throat tightened; my eyes watered. *She's dying*, I thought. *She's dying*. I felt woozy and reached behind me for a chair. I sat with my head between my knees for a few minutes and then looked up. Jane was still there, still intubated, still unconscious.

I sat in that chair, staring at Jane, wondering what our future would look like or whether we'd even have one. If she didn't survive, I would be devastated. But if she did survive—hardly a sure thing—I'd have to care for her. I had no idea what that might involve. Would she be crippled by heart or lung damage? Had her brain been deprived of oxygen for too long? And, if by some miracle, she survived intact, how long would it be before her breast cancer killed her? One year? Two years? No more, certainly, not with that CT picture. Would I have the strength to do this?

Then, I surprised myself: along with these worries I felt the first stirrings of long-suppressed anger and resentment toward Jane. Why had she been so cagey with me about her breast cancer—hinting at half-truths and refusing my help? She seemed to trust me in all other aspects of our lives. Why was this different? I asked myself these questions over and over in a variety of unproductive ways for the next two hours.

It was now close to midnight. Since noon, I'd been running at the highest emotional pitch I'd ever experienced and was ready to collapse. I desperately needed a few hours of normalcy, something that would give me a chance to regroup and gather strength for what was to come. A night in my own bed, however brief, could help. But the mere thought made me feel unforgivably selfish. A good husband would sit at his wife's bedside for the duration, head propped up, dozing intermittently.

I just couldn't do it, so I went out to talk to the head nurse. I sheepishly said that I had to go home and try to grab a few hours of sleep. Would that be all right? I think my actual words were, "Would that be terrible of me?"

Without waiting for an answer I might not want to hear, I gave her my cell number and told her she should have a very low threshold for calling me if anything changed—I could be back in ten minutes. I can't remember how the nurse looked at me. Was it really with disdain or was I projecting? She probably reassured me, but I have no memory of that.

I went back into Jane's room. I looked at her for a few more minutes, then kissed her on the forehead and walked out of the ICU.

THREE

I slept fitfully for a few hours—no calls from the ICU, thank goodness—and woke without an alarm around six. I sat on the edge of the bed, aware that I was alone. I thought about how my Saturdays used to begin by bringing Jane her breakfast and realized I wouldn't be doing that today. Is this what life would be like from now on? It felt horrible.

I showered, dressed, and drove back to the hospital. I walked a roundabout route from the parking lot to the ICU, bypassing the passenger elevators—I wasn't ready to run into anyone I knew. I assumed that people would have heard about Jane by now and I was afraid that I'd lose my composure if someone were to ask me about her.

Everything felt unreal, dreamlike. *Am I really on my way to visit my dying wife in intensive care?* I kept thinking that this couldn't possibly be happening. But it was. As I entered the ICU, I glanced down the hall toward the open door of Jane's room. There she was— still unconscious, still intubated, Propofol still running through her IV line.

I stopped at the nursing station to ask how her night had been. It had been quiet, I was told, and her vital signs were now stable. That was good news, but I knew the outlook was still grim.

I took a deep breath and walked into Jane's room. A flimsy curtain hung from a rod over the doorway. I drew it closed in a vain attempt to give us some privacy and sat down next to the bed. It was easier this morning to look at her face, which was placid and still beautiful despite the breathing tube in her mouth. I leaned over and kissed her on her forehead. I put my mouth close to her ear and told her that she'd had a large pulmonary embolus and was now on a ventilator in the ICU but that she was getting better. I told her that I loved her very much. I knew that Jane was unconscious and couldn't hear me—I'm a realist—but talking to her made her seem more alive and felt like a kind thing to do.

I sat back in the chair. I didn't want to read the book I had brought; I didn't want to watch television.

* * *

"Do you understand my role here?"

Whenever Jane told our origin story, she claimed that these were the first words I spoke to her. She insisted that they were accompanied by a patronizing sneer.

In April 1983, I was a senior resident in my final year of internal medicine training at Boston's Beth Israel Hospital. My job that month was to oversee two inpatient teams, one led by me and the other by a junior resident. Each team was made up of three first-year interns, and each intern was responsible for eight to ten patients. Beth Israel is a Harvard teaching hospital, so each team also had a medical student doing a mandatory three-month "rotation" to learn about internal medicine. A new group of students had just started. Jane had been assigned to the junior resident's team; a different student had been assigned to mine.

Every three days I had to work a thirty-six-hour shift, which meant an overnight stay in the hospital. On those nights "on call," one of my responsibilities was to determine which patients on the regular wards were sick enough to be transferred to the ICU. On Jane's second day in the hospital, which happened to coincide with one of my long shifts, her resident told her to swing by the ICU to check on the status of a patient their team had transferred the day before.

It was late afternoon and, in anticipation of my night's work, I had stopped by the ICU to see how many slots were available. As I walked around the unit counting empty beds, I looked up to see a beautiful, willowy woman making her way toward me. Even in the ridiculous-looking short white coat that students were forced to wear, she was stunning.

Although Jane would later be known as the master of every situation, that day she looked lost. I can't remember exactly what she asked, but I do remember thinking that her question was odd and betrayed some confusion about how things worked in the ICU. A new medical student's unfamiliarity with the mechanics of hospital life would be excusable and the ICU was an especially complicated place. The problem was that Jane had posed her question to someone who couldn't answer it: me. I thought she would be better served by one of the interns, residents, or nurses who were actually running the unit. I was just passing through. Not wanting to seem dismissive, I tried to ease into my response by asking if she understood my role. Wrong question, apparently.

Regardless of what I may have said at that first meeting or how I may have said it, we both felt something electric—the first spark of what became an irresistible mutual attraction. Over the next month, despite the decidedly unromantic milieu of the hospital, we devised ingenious ways to flirt with each other. Some required detailed planning. My favorite involved the fact that medical students were expected to analyze urine samples from their patients. Jane knew that the only microscope available for this purpose was in the emergency room. She also knew that another of my responsibilities as a senior resident was to help in the emergency room as needed. So, Jane kept tabs on my whereabouts, and whenever I was in the ER, she scrambled to find a patient whose urine she could examine. After several days coming up dry, she decided to take matters into her own hands. She peed into a specimen cup and brought it to the ER, pretending it was from a patient. Her stratagem worked. I ran into her in the microscope room, where we talked and flirted.

For my part, I looked for ways to sit next to Jane in conferences so that I could amuse her with whispered running commentaries. I'm quite sure that no one would have found me as entertaining as I did, but who cares? It was an excuse for us to be near each other. Or, if I saw Jane standing at a nursing station writing a note in a patient's medical chart, it would suddenly occur to me that I, too, had to write a note, and the most convenient place to do so would just happen to be that narrow space right next to her. While writing our notes, we would "accidentally" brush hands. It was exhilarating.

I was smitten and wanted to ask her out, but the thought made me uneasy. By the time I'd met Jane, I was already the veteran of a short-lived starter marriage that hadn't survived my residency and I'd been divorced for about a year. My failed marriage did produce one great success: my daughter, Anna, who then was four years old and the light of my life. Some of my discomfort about dating Jane could have come from the difficulties I imagined I'd have as a single father trying to start a new romance.

But that wasn't it. Instead, my hesitation arose directly from an understanding of my professional position. The power differential between a resident and a medical student is huge, and a liaison between someone like me and someone like Jane would not be tolerated today—rightly so. Even back in those benighted times, when a resident could pursue a student with impunity, I was uncomfortable about the idea that I might be exploiting my position in the medical hierarchy. So, to assuage my guilt, I marshalled several marginally relevant facts. First, Jane was on the *other* team, so I had no direct role in evaluating her performance; second, she had spent several years on a different career path before going to medical school and was now thirty-one years old, exactly my age, so I wouldn't be robbing the cradle; third, in just a few months, she would rotate off the medical service. I admit that these facts did nothing to get me off the ethical hook, but I clung to them just the same.

Armed with these rationalizations, I asked Jane out. My dating strategy was to impress her by taking her to restaurants recommended by my more worldly friends—I presumed they'd point me toward reasonably good places. I imagined that Jane and I would linger over coffee, talking deep into the evening, and that my dazzling conversational skills would make her fall in love with me.

Jane had other ideas. She did let me take her to dinner but as soon as the main course was cleared, she said that she was tired and needed to go home. I paid the bill and dutifully drove her home thinking that I'd just had a failed date. But when we got to her apartment, Jane didn't want me to drop her off. She told me to find a place to park and come inside. This happened on each of our first three dates. Sometimes her invitation would lead to sex. Other times, we'd just sit in front of the TV. Both outcomes were eminently satisfying, believe it or not.

After our third date, while we were sitting on her bed, fully clothed and watching some forgettable sitcom, Jane turned to me and spoke.

"I just thought you should know," she said in a flat, undramatic tone, "I'm going to marry you."

That should have freaked me out, but it didn't; it made me happy. I had just started to understand what Jane already knew—we were meant for each other.

The path to relationship heaven, however, is seldom smooth or straight. In addition to the problem created by the mismatch in our professional positions, there was the small matter of Jane's current boyfriend, a professor at the medical school. Although the magnitude of their power differential dwarfed ours, I couldn't use that information to ease my conscience because I didn't know about it. Jane took her sweet time before saying anything to me—we had already been dating for a month before she casually mentioned that she had been stepping out on the professor. To be fair, the relationship had soured, but it was still ongoing, and I think Jane saw me as a means to extricate herself.

The soon-to-be ex did not go quietly. First, he tortured Jane. He let himself into her apartment using the key she had given him in rosier times and cut himself out of photos of the two of them together. He bought her a subscription to *Playboy*. He signed her up for the Pantyhose-of-the-Month Club— size XX-Large. Then he tortured me. He got someone in her class to leave an anonymous typed note in my mailbox at the hospital. I still remember what it said:

Dr. Rollins:

Harvard medical students at the Beth Israel Hospital are there for medical rather than sexual education. Using your position as a resident to take advantage of such a student was a flagrant violation of your status. It will be remembered here at the Beth Israel and other Harvard-affiliated institutions.

This was a risky move considering how flagrantly he had been violating his own status as a professor.

The final bump in the road came right before Jane broke up with him. We had been invited to a fireworks viewing party on July 4, a last hurrah for me since I was starting my fellowship at Dana-Farber the next day. Jane told me she would meet me at the party, but she never showed. I called her apartment several times—no answer. Worried sick in those pre–cell phone days, I went home and sat by the old rotary hoping it would ring. Finally, at around midnight, I tried calling again. This time, Jane picked up.

"Hello?" she said.

"It's me," I said quickly.

"Hi," she said with a casualness that belied the circumstances.

"Yeah, hi, I guess," I said, starting to feel more confused than worried. "Where were you? I've spent the past five hours thinking that something horrible had happened."

"Oh, really?" she replied. "No, I'm fine. I'm sorry if I made you worry. How was the party?"

"The party may have been great," I said. "I don't actually know because I was so distracted by your failure to show and then my concern when you didn't. What happened?"

"I just lost track of the time," she said. "Again, I'm so sorry."

"Come on," I said. "You weren't home. I called a dozen times."

"I was at Nathaniel's house," she said flatly. That was her professor boyfriend.

"You're kidding," I said.

"No. I went over there to break up with him," she said.

That was welcome news.

"I'm glad you decided to make it definitive," I said, somewhat mollified. "How'd it go?"

"Well, I gathered up all of the stuff from my place that I thought he could possibly want—there wasn't very much, to tell the truth—and took it over to his house. When he let me in, I dumped it all on his dining room table and told him we were breaking up."

"Very direct," I said. "Good for you. How'd he take it?"

"Well, he tried to convince me that we could work things out, that he could change all of the things that I'd been finding so obnoxious and irritating, including his recent psychotic behavior. But I told him I was having none of it."

"Again, good for you," I said. "But that shouldn't have taken very long."

"Well, he kept on pleading and I kept on saying no. So, eventually we had breakup sex. I only got home about ten minutes ago."

I was flabbergasted.

"Wait!" I said. "What about us? What about this great life we've been planning together? You said you wanted to marry me."

"I still do. I love you," she said.

"But you just fucked your old boyfriend!" I was nearly shouting.

"Well, yeah," she said. "But it was breakup sex."

"What *is* that?" I said. "Whatever it is, you can't use it an excuse for cheating on me."

"I wasn't cheating on you," she said with some vehemence. "Haven't you ever heard of breakup sex?"

"Evidently, I've led a sheltered life," I replied. "And even if there were such a thing, it still doesn't excuse your behavior."

"Well, there is such a thing," she said. "And it ended my relationship with Nathaniel. I am totally committed to you and want to marry you."

"Even putting the sex aside," I said, not wanting to let Jane know that she'd partially pacified me, "you didn't call me for five hours to let me know that you were okay."

I was very aware that I sounded like my mother, but I didn't want to give up my anger yet.

"You're right," Jane said. "I'm sorry about that too. I won't ever let that happen again."

"I have to think about all of this," I said. "I also have to go to sleep. My fellowship starts tomorrow and I can't stay up 'til all hours talking about this tonight."

"I understand," she said. "Call me tomorrow."

"Good night," I said and hung up.

I was pretty angry. I refused to call Jane for a week. Eventually, I calmed down and found myself thinking about all the things I loved about her. I knew I still wanted to be with her. And, after all, she had just made a clean, albeit sexualized, break with her old boyfriend. This episode might well have been festooned with bright red warning flags—plus sirens and flashing lights—but I didn't see them. I was too far gone to let it keep us apart. I relented and, from that moment on, we were inseparable.

* * *

I was still thinking about breakup sex when a nurse came in to check on Jane's IV lines.

"How are we both doing?" she asked.

I recognized Colleen from yesterday but hadn't seen her yet today. She must have just started her shift. She reminded me of all the tough, no-nonsense ICU nurses I had worked with when I was a resident. She was Irish, had a thick South Boston accent you could cut with a knife, and was kind of scary but totally on our team.

"Hanging in, I guess," I replied.

"Well, it looks like Jane's been pretty stable, so that's a very good thing," she said. "I'm just going to take a peek at her IV sites to make sure everything's still flowing as it should and that nothing looks infected."

As the nurse lifted Jane's left hand to get a better look at the IV, a sparkle caught my eye. It was the overhead light glinting off of Jane's wedding ring. I looked at it and laughed.

A few months into our relationship, after the business with her old boyfriend had been put behind us, Jane asked me to describe the wedding ring I had given my first wife. It was an antique diamond in a platinum setting that had belonged to my grandmother. After the divorce, my ex-wife, who knew the ring's provenance and its sentimental value, generously returned it.

Jane asked if she could see it. I retrieved the ring from the freezer in the kitchen where I had cleverly been hiding it from robbers. Jane picked it up, telling me how beautiful it was, and slipped it on the fourth finger of her left hand. She looked at it admiringly for a minute or two.

"Okay, let's put it back on ice," I said.

"No, I don't think so," she said. "I'm keeping it right where it is."

I laughed, but she was serious. It remained on her finger until the day she died.

This was, in retrospect, an unexpected commitment because I was not at all certain that Jane and I would ever be married, despite what she had said on date three. It's not that we weren't devoted to each other—we were. Almost from the start, I spent most nights at Jane's apartment in Cambridge and we soon made a more formal decision to live together. Based on a tip from one of Jane's friends, we found a great apartment in Brookline, only ten minutes from the hospitals where we worked. That's where we began our official cohabitation.

After moving in, we did try to fulfill Jane's prophecy that we would get married. Jane only had about six months of medical school left to go and she was sure she'd be able to manage a wedding right after she finished school. Of course, the timing was ridiculously impractical. She would graduate in June and her internship—a notoriously time-consuming and unforgiving ordeal—would begin in July. Still, as medical school wound down, she started to plan an August wedding and even found a dress. I tried to be helpful but kept pointing out that her internship was looming and that it would be a miracle if she were able to find time to sleep, much less get married. She dismissed my concerns.

But by the second week of July, with her internship well under-way, Jane could see that there would be no August wedding. Fortunately, she was too exhausted to be disappointed. At that point, we decided just to get on with our lives, figuring that things would eventually quiet down long enough for us to get married.

That finally happened nine years later. By then, Jane and I had been taking regular week-long vacations on Nantucket where we'd rent a house and spend our days reading or going to the beach. Jane had decided, rather arbitrarily, that she did not want a large wedding and was not interested in inviting any relatives to a ceremony on the island. I'm not sure where her aversion came from but she seemed to be acting on a principle she once described to one of her trainees, a young woman who had breathlessly told Jane about the gigantic wedding she was planning, replete with multiple dress changes, horses, and an audience of four hundred.

"You know, Megha," Jane said, cocking her head to one side. "Big weddings are for little girls."

Jane was a big girl and was determined to have a minuscule wedding.

We completed all the blood and license work in Boston, and I found a justice of the peace in Nantucket who was willing to perform the ceremony. On the appointed day, Jane put on a flowing plum-colored pantsuit that she had chosen for the occasion—her one concession to the special nature of the event—and I drove us to the justice's house.

We were greeted at the door by a plethoric woman in her sixties with dyed dirty-blond hair. A cigarette dangled from one corner of her mouth.

"Hi there, kids," she said with a rasp that would put Wolfman Jack to shame. "Come on in. Let's get you married."

We followed her into the living room where she planted herself in front of an empty fireplace. She indicated that Jane and I were to stand facing her.

"One minute," she said as she stubbed out her cigarette in the ashtray on the mantle and lit up a fresh one.

"Okay," she said, taking a long drag. "What else, what else.... Oh, yeah. Herb!" she shouted over her shoulder.

"What?" said a male voice from another room.

"I need you in the living room," she said.

"What for?" Herb shouted.

"I need a witness. Get in here pronto."

Herb ambled into the living room wiping crumbs from his mouth with a napkin.

"I was having lunch," he whined.

"It'll keep," croaked his wife. "This won't take long."

The justice turned to us, gave the usual preamble, and had us repeat our vows. Jane had taken off my grandmother's ring so I could put it back on her fourth finger. Which I did. There was no ring for me. We were declared man and wife.

The justice signed the marriage license, Herb went back to his lunch, and we left. The rest of the vacation was our honeymoon.

As it turned out, Jane hadn't told her mother that she was getting married. I'm pretty sure that her mother never forgave her for getting married on the sly.

However, our colleagues at work knew about the wedding. So, Jane returned to an office decorated with silver streamers attached to the ceiling lights, several vases of cut flowers, and a huge sign congratulating us. The people who worked for Jane loved her despite her occasional lapses into meanness like the snide comment about big weddings and little girls.

These memories seemed disconnected from the woman lying in the bed fighting for her life and the man who was sitting by her side watching her. I waited until Colleen left the room, then picked up Jane's left hand. I stared at her ring and gave it one full turn around her finger, just to make sure it wasn't too tight.

It occurred to me that if Jane were to die, someone would have to remove the ring from her finger and give it to me. I'd probably put the ring back in its box in the freezer. For thirty years, Jane would have only been borrowing it.

FOUR

I was roused from my reveries by the ICU team on their morning rounds, the time-honored practice of visiting each patient in turn to hear about how they'd fared overnight and to develop a plan for the coming day. The team had reached Jane's room and were hovering at the door, awaiting permission to enter. As I stood to acknowledge their presence, the scrum tumbled across the threshold. Along with Tony, the ICU chief from last night, were his resident, two interns, a respiratory therapist, a pharmacist, and two nurses.

"She had a quiet night," Tony began, addressing me. "Her numbers are improving and her blood pressure is stable. Things seem to be going in the right direction but I do want to get a CT-angio today or tomorrow to see for sure that the clot has been dissolved."

"Okay, thanks," I said. "That's great news. When can Jane come off the ventilator?"

"Oh, oh, not for a while yet," he replied, shaking his head. "She still needs very high levels of oxygen. It'll take days to wean her off the vent."

While Tony spoke, the other members of the team focused their attention on the monitors over Jane's head, engrossed by the steady stream of data—heart rate, blood pressure, oxygen levels. Then, like a flock of birds wheeling synchronously in response to a signal only they could sense, the team pivoted as one and left the room. Tony started to follow but stopped at the door. He turned toward me.

"The, um, mass is bleeding," he said in a low voice. "We need to bring in a surgeon to look at it. Would that be all right?"

Tony was trying to be sensitive about my request to limit the number of people who knew about Jane's cancer. I appreciated his concern but wasn't too worried. A surgeon with the right expertise might have some kind of adjunct appointment at the Farber but would be employed at the Brigham, away from Jane's friends and coworkers.

"Yes, of course. By all means," I said.

Tony nodded and scurried out of the room to catch up with his team, which had moved on to their next patient.

I resumed my seat next to Jane. How odd this all was. The team's discomfort had been palpable, and I thought I understood why. The medical hierarchy—Germanic in its rigidity and intricate taxonomy—was deeply embedded in teaching hospitals like the Brigham. This morning's patient, a mortally ill woman with what appeared to be a neglected breast cancer, was technically their superior. She was a Professor of Medicine at Harvard Medical School who had been the team leader's teacher. They must have been struggling to find the right way to deal with her as a patient.

Their unease had to do with their understanding of Jane's status—her position at the very pinnacle of the medical world. Of course, she hadn't suddenly appeared there, fully armed like Athena. She was a midwestern girl whose path to medicine had actually been anything but straightforward. In fact, Jane had majored in philosophy as an undergrad at Harvard College and had given no thought to what she'd do after graduation. The path of least resistance was to follow her boyfriend to Washington, DC, where he'd used an inheritance to start an art gallery. After an aimless year working with him, she landed a clerical position at the Urban Institute, a liberal think tank. Within a few months, her smarts got her noticed and she was assigned to a project evaluating Medicare and Medicaid policies for nursing homes.

To her surprise, Jane found that she enjoyed this kind of policy work and was good at it. After a few years, she decided that the best way to turn her interest into a career would be to go to law school. Her older brother, Tom, was a lawyer, so this path was familiar. Jane applied to law schools and was accepted by several. She chose Harvard.

Before matriculating, however, two things happened. First, she saw the movie *The Paper Chase*. Its depiction of the life of a first-year law student scared the daylights out of her. Second, she met a woman at a party who happened to be a doctor. In the course of their conversation, Jane mentioned her health policy work and her doubts about law school. The woman pointed out that doctors also do health policy work and asked Jane if she had considered medical school instead. When Jane said that this was an impossible choice because she hadn't taken any science courses in college, the woman laughed. She herself had made a late-life decision to become a doctor and had fulfilled all the course requirements for medical school in a post-baccalaureate program.

The next day, Jane asked Harvard Law School to defer her admission for a year. Once her request was granted, she moved back to Cambridge and enrolled in Harvard's post-bac program. She also worked a variety of jobs to support herself. It was an extraordinarily time-consuming effort that precluded any social life. Instead of friends, her constant companions were her records. In particular, she developed an unusual affinity for Elvis Costello—she played his albums over and over until she wore them out. Years later, while reminiscing about this time, Jane said, "I know it can't possibly be true but there's something about Elvis's voice that makes me think he's talking directly to me. Does that make me sound crazy?"

I said that it didn't but my answer was tentative.

Jane performed well in her courses. When the time came for her to apply to medical school, she withdrew from Harvard Law, sent in her med school applications, and was accepted at several. Of course, she chose Harvard.

When Jane started medical school in 1980, she was twenty-eight, older than the majority of her classmates, most of whom had gone straight to medical school after college. The few students who were closer to her age all found each other and formed a clique that didn't mix much with the younger students. For some reason, none of those friendships lasted beyond medical school. I can't remember socializing with any of Jane's classmates in later years. This was her usual practice—Jane hadn't kept any friends from high school or college either.

By the time we met, Jane had only one more year of medical school to go. Internship and residency would be next, which meant that she would have to choose a medical specialty—there are different residencies for different specialties like surgery, obstetrics, internal medicine, and so on. Jane was a born internist. Specialists in internal medicine often can't do anything to make a patient better but they sure love arguing about it. Endlessly. That fit her like a glove.

Later, at the end of residency, Jane decided that she wanted to subspecialize in a specific area of internal medicine. She chose oncology. I think she liked the fact that cancer had become the most complex field in medicine, and she thought that she could make a real contribution. That meant she would have to endure at least four more years of training in a fellowship program. Through my experiences at Dana-Farber, Jane had a good understanding of how that institution worked. She liked the idea of training there—it was another Harvard program, after all—so she applied to the fellowship and was accepted. Not surprisingly, she did a great job and was recruited to join the faculty in 1992. So began our twenty-year run of lunches together.

* * *

I was rudely yanked out of the past again, this time by a respiratory therapist who was using a loud suction apparatus to remove mucus from the tube in Jane's throat. Her situation was so medically complex. I thought for a moment about the daunting fact that she was only one of a dozen patients in the ICU, each with their own set of intricate problems.

It had been twenty-four hours since Jane's collapse. She'd been desperately ill since then, looking like she was about to die at any moment. I'd been watching it all, terrified about the future. I needed to talk to someone—someone who could share my anxiety or, better, to reassure me that Jane would be fine. But I had no one.

Jane was not close to her family, nor was I particularly close to mine. I didn't feel like I could lean on them for support. For years, Jane and I had led a hermetic existence, relying exclusively on each other for companionship and support.

But I did need to let Jane's family know how ill she was. This was hardly a straightforward matter because, for as long as we'd been together, Jane had kept her family at bay. Contact was sporadic at best, and she rarely talked about them. Although her studied indifference was directed toward her family as a whole, her feelings about specific members ran the gamut from admiration to apathy to disdain.

Tales from Jane's childhood suggested that she'd enjoyed a close relationship with her father, an English professor at the University of Michigan. Jane's verbal skills and intellect manifested at an early age, which endeared her to his professorial side. But he'd also been an army medic during World War II with thwarted dreams of becoming a doctor, so her decision to go to medical school gave him a vicarious way to experience his deferred ambition through his favorite child. Or so Jane told me.

Although never quite explicit in their details, stories from Jane and other family members hinted at a physical intimacy with her father that bordered on the inappropriate. I had seen them together during Christmas visits to her childhood home in Ann Arbor, and it was true that their relationship did occasionally incline toward the creepy. Nothing shocking, just unsettling vignettes like Jane moaning quasi-sexually while her dad rubbed her feet. Maybe it was all fine and only seemed jarring in comparison to my own father's icy remoteness. Mostly, though, her father seemed to be in thrall to his daughter—more than she was to him.

Jane's father died of prostate cancer a few years after I'd met him. It happened while Jane was a resident at the Brigham and, despite her grueling schedule, she figured out a way to spend several weeks with him in Ann Arbor while he was dying. More evidence of their closeness.

Jane's older brother, Tom, was a lawyer who ran a legal aid office in Ohio. Although Jane admired him, nearly all her stories involved Tom's exercise of a big brother's God-given right to torture his little sister. These were funny, kid-stuff anecdotes—teasing Jane for her inability to drive (he called her "Parnelli Jane") or forcing her into logical quagmires of the "Why are you hitting yourself" variety. The odd thing was how compulsively Jane would resurrect her resentments during our Christmas visits, usually accompanied by complaints that their mother hadn't reined Tom in. Jane invested a lot of psychic energy in seeking belated justice.

Although she appeared incapable of resolving her childhood feelings about Tom, the two of them eventually developed a meaningful adult relationship. She never called him—actually, Jane never initiated contact with anybody—but she would happily talk for an hour or more whenever he called her.

Jane had trouble achieving even this level of intimacy with her younger sister, Sarah. For reasons I'll never understand, Jane looked down on her. Sarah was talented and creative—she became a bestselling author of children's books and YA fiction—but those weren't attributes that Jane respected. She looked for intellect and academic achievement. Plus, Sarah competed with Jane for her father's affections. Altogether a bad combination. We only saw Sarah at Christmas and rarely had contact at other times.

Despite all this distancing, Jane seemed to melt when her siblings had children of their own. Both had two boys apiece, and Jane was fascinated by her nephews. She kept framed pictures and looked forward to spending time with them during our Christmas visits when she assumed the role of the cool, trouble-making aunt. One year, she had us buy a plastic Uzi for Tom's older son, Bill. Jane sat back with an evil smile as Bill, after opening his present, ran around the living room shooting his gun and driving his parents crazy.

Later, Jane was deeply invested in the academic career of Brian, Bill's younger brother. He was in a graduate program in evolutionary biology and Jane enthusiastically gave advice—either directly or through Tom—about writing research papers and framing their arguments for maximum impact.

I've saved Jane's mother for last. Fran is a loving woman utterly devoted to all her children. I emphasize her devotion to all because Jane didn't make it easy to be included in the maternal embrace. This tension was on full display during Christmas. On one hand, despite Jane's emotional distance from her family, she could be totally engaged in holiday events. On Christmas morning, for example, she would insist that she be "Santa" and hand out presents according to an arcane algorithm known only to her. While this might have been an endearing display of childlike behavior, what she really loved was being in the spotlight and controlling the flow of the morning's events. Jane was also an enthusiastic player of the games—Pictionary, Trivial Pursuit, Monopoly—that took up the rest of our time, and which she usually won.

On the other hand, Jane barely interacted with her mother. No offers to help with cooking, no shopping for meals, and only perfunctory gestures toward setting the table or cleaning up. Fran would try to engage Jane in conversation about her life in Boston, and Jane, while never rude or sullen, would offer minimal responses. My auditory memory of those visits is Fran beginning every conversation with a beseeching, "Honey...?" which was answered by monosyllables.

"Honey...how's work?"

"Okay."

"Are you teaching much?"

"No, not at all."

"Oh. So, what are you doing?"

"Research."

"That's exciting. What are you studying?"

"It's complicated."

"But do you like it? Are you enjoying it?"

"Yeah, sure."

Why did Jane seem to have so little respect for her mother? Was it because of that priority she placed on intellect and academic achievement? Was it because of intrafamilial rivalry—she was her father's daughter while Tom was her mother's son? (I'm not sure where that left Sarah.) I don't know, but the outcome was tragic. Fran never gave up trying to connect with Jane, and Jane never gave her satisfaction.

* * *

Now I had to let Jane's family—all of them—know that she was in the ICU, but what could I tell them about why she was there? Most people would find comfort in sharing a cancer diagnosis with their loved ones, but not Jane. She had been hiding her breast cancer from everyone, and I had to assume that she had included her family among the ignorant and would want to keep it that way. But really, how could I tell them she was in intensive care without mentioning the disease that was killing her? I am very loyal, but I am also a terrible liar. I decided to help Jane keep her secret, but I resented the fact that her secrecy had put me in this bind.

I walked to the hallway outside the ICU and called Jane's sister.

"Sarah, I have terrible news. Jane became very ill yesterday and she's now in intensive care."

39

"Oh, my god," Sarah cried. "What happened? Is she dying? Should I be there?"

I told Sarah that Jane had a massive blood clot in her chest which made it difficult for her heart to pump blood and for her lungs to provide oxygen to her body. I said that she had experienced something like a cardiac arrest and that she now needed a machine to help her breathe. Fortunately, she had been given a drug to break up the clot and it looked like it was working.

There. I'd done it, and I hadn't told a single lie.

"But why did this happen?"

Crap. Now I'd have to lie. The whole reason for Jane's pulmonary embolus was her underlying disease—patients with widespread cancer have a propensity to form blood clots. I knew I'd have to commit a sin of omission.

"We don't know," I lied, with a confidence that surprised me. "The doctors are looking for a cause but their first priority is to get her heart and lungs stabilized."

I felt terrible. I knew Sarah would have wanted to know about Jane's cancer but I also knew that Jane wouldn't have wanted me to tell her. I could only hope that Sarah would forgive me when she eventually learned the truth. I told her that there was no need to come to Boston yet and that I'd keep her informed about Jane's status. She reluctantly agreed to stay home.

Then I called Tom. The conversation was almost identical to the one I'd had with Sarah except that the lying came a little more easily. Even so, there was a hint of skepticism in Tom's voice. I don't think he fully bought the story. That was the lawyer in him.

By the time I talked to Jane's mother, the lies had become second nature.

"Oh, Jane! Poor Jane!" Fran said when I told her about her daughter's pulmonary embolus and being intubated in the ICU. "I have to be there. She needs me."

"I understand," I said. "But, Fran, she's unconscious and wouldn't know that you're here."

"But she needs me," Fran repeated.

"I think she does, Fran," I said, trying to be sympathetic. "But it would be a very difficult trip for you."

Fran was ninety-four years old and suffering from bad hip pain. Getting on a plane to Boston would not be easy for her.

"Let's wait a few days," I continued, "and see how things are going. Jane's already better today than she was yesterday. If she continues to improve and wake up, then it might be better for you to make the effort when she actually knows you're here."

"I suppose," Fran said quietly. "I just wish I could help her right now."

"I don't blame you," I said. "But there's really nothing that any of us can do who aren't her doctors."

"Yes, I can see that," she said.

Fran paused.

"Why do you think this happened?" she asked.

There it was. My cue to dodge, weave, and lie.

"We really don't know, Fran. People can get these blood clots for all sorts of reasons. The important thing is that it's being treated in one of the best hospitals in the world and Jane's getting better."

"Yes, yes. That's comforting," she said. "Jane's so lucky to have you there with her."

"She's lucky that she has great doctors and such a loving family," I said. "I promise to keep you and Tom and Sarah updated constantly. You'll know right away if anything happens."

My queasiness at misleading Jane's family, especially her mother, was tempered by relief that I'd kept her secret.

FIVE

Returning to Jane's room in the ICU, I found a woman dressed in surgical scrubs bending over Jane, listening to her heart and lungs. She straightened up when she saw me, took the stethoscope out of her ears, and introduced herself. Sue was the surgeon the ICU team had called. Her short, blonde bob framed a kind face.

We exchanged pleasantries. Then, with a smile, Sue said, "Okay, let's see what we have here."

She reached behind me to close the curtain over the doorway and then gingerly pulled down the top of Jane's hospital gown. This was the first time I had taken a close look at the mass. It was truly horrific. Far bigger than the breast it had replaced, it rose six or seven inches above Jane's chest. It was black—the technical term is necrotic—with an irregular, bumpy surface. Deep holes pierced it at random intervals; some oozed blood, others pus. The whole thing had a wet sheen caused by a serum-like liquid it exuded. The normal skin at the mass's margins was bright red; it looked inflamed, maybe infected. Satellite growths had popped up in the skin a few inches away from the main mass. The largest cluster, about a half dozen in number, marched in a line across Jane's upper chest toward her neck.

Again, my grip tightened around the railing on the side of Jane's bed—a familiar wooziness was making its presence known. I have a profound, exaggeratedly visceral response to this kind of grotesque distortion of the human body, especially when it's caused by disease.

I couldn't control my reaction—it was like a reflex—and I was deeply ashamed of it. I was worried that this weakness would make me incapable of caring for my wife. That humiliating thought had occurred to me the day before, when I'd caught my first glimpse of the mass in the emergency room. Now I was convinced that a closer inspection would simply overwhelm me. I'd never fainted before. Would this be the first time?

What happened instead was that looking at the tumor with Sue had a calming effect. I kept one eye on the mass but the other was on Sue as she examined it, prodding here and there with her gloved hands. Her movements were accompanied by a quiet narration.

"Looks like a little bleeding there," she murmured softly to herself. "I can take care of that. Looks like this area might be infected; we can culture some of that. Looks like there's a lot of weepy liquid; we can figure out how to make a dressing to absorb that."

Sue assessed the tumor without betraying a hint of shock or disgust—her attention was focused on formulating a plan to manage it. Watching her quiet competence made all the difference. She gave me a way of looking objectively at the cancer without objectifying Jane.

Sue took a tiny biopsy of the tumor near its edge where there seemed to be more living tissue. This would be sent to the pathologists, who would officially make the diagnosis of breast cancer that everyone, starting with Jane, had unofficially made. Then Sue carefully dressed the mass the way a surgeon would dress a wound. This was a learning experience for me. She made me smile at one point when she folded small pieces of gauze and stuffed them into some of the mass's deeper crevices.

"We call these flowers," she said.

When she finished, she replaced Jane's gown and turned to me.

"So, who's Jane's oncologist?" she asked.

"Eric," I replied.

Sue smiled. She and Eric had worked together for years.

"That's great. I think he's out of town, but I'll talk to him when he's back," said Sue.

"Thanks," I said. "Please do. But there's one more favor I need to ask."

I was starting to sound like a broken record.

"Jane has told no one about her breast cancer. You, Eric, and the ICU team are the only people who know about it. I realize that the information will eventually come out one way or another but, for now, could I ask you to keep it confidential?"

Without hesitating, Sue said, "Yes, of course. No worries."

Her professionalism was comforting. I gave her a lot of credit for pretending that this was a routine medical situation and that my absurd request was perfectly reasonable.

Sue left. I kissed Jane softly on the forehead, whispered goodbye, and headed for home to spend my second night alone. I felt like I had spent my whole day finding ways to accommodate Jane's outrageous secrecy about her cancer. Why? Why had she made an inherently impossible situation even more difficult?

* * *

After three decades of living with Jane, I had become adept at adjusting to her quirky behaviors. None was more deeply embedded than her aversion to seeking medical care for herself. In all the years I knew her, she never had a primary care doctor and never went to a routine medical appointment. She had one root canal when her tooth pain became unbearable but, other than that, she never went to a dentist or a hygienist. She suffered for years from intense lower back pain and sciatica but never sought help. Despite working in, and eventually leading, a world-class academic center devoted to cancer screening and prevention, she never had a single mammogram, Pap smear, or colonoscopy.

Sometimes the consequences of her stubbornness could be alarming. About fifteen years earlier, Jane started having recurring attacks of excruciating abdominal pain and fever. I worried that she might have diverticulitis or worse. But no matter what I said, I could not convince her to see a doctor. Instead, she called our drugstore to prescribe herself a powerful antibiotic and asked me to pick it up for her. Sometimes this strategy worked, and she would recover after a few days. Other times the first antibiotic didn't do the trick and she would prescribe herself a second one. During one protracted episode, she missed several weeks of work while she lay in bed, waiting to see if she would get better. She eventually did, and life went on.

I don't know where Jane's intense medical phobias came from, but they had dire results. They were, in fact, the direct cause of the misery she was now experiencing.

One Saturday morning about four years before the pulmonary embolism, I heard Jane calling to me from behind the closed door of our bathroom. I opened it to find a horrific sight. Jane was lying on the tile floor. The caftan she wore on weekends was partially unzipped and over her right shoulder was a blood-soaked towel.

"My god!" I nearly shouted. "What's wrong?"

"I'm dying," she said calmly.

"What are you talking about?" I asked, skeptical but concerned about her uncharacteristically dramatic assertion.

"I have breast cancer," she said.

"Really?" I said, still skeptical. "How do you know?"

Jane didn't reply. She continued to lie on the floor, looking any-where but my direction.

I let a minute pass.

"Seriously, hon," I said in a softer tone. "What's this about?"

Again, no reply.

"Look," I said, "I can't help you if you won't tell me what's happening."

"Fine," she said, with a note of disgust creeping into her voice. "I have breast cancer that's spread to my skin. It's invaded a blood vessel and now I'm bleeding to death."

"Jesus Christ! Let me see how serious this is," I said, reaching for the zipper.

"No!" she screamed. "Don't touch me! I just don't want to be alone when I die."

"How do you know you're dying?" I said. "How do you even know this is breast cancer?"

"Oh, I am and it is."

"Well, I can't just let you die here on the floor," I said, reaching for my phone. "I'm calling 911."

"No, no, no!" she screamed again. "Don't you dare. *I'll never forgive you if you do.*"

I froze. I was utterly loyal to Jane but this behavior was insane. We sat in silence for a few more minutes.

"Why don't you read to me?" she finally said. She'd brought the *New York Times* into the bathroom. It was lying on the floor next to her, so I picked it up and started reading aloud.

After an hour, Jane still wasn't dead.

"I think the bleeding stopped," she said.

"Thank god," I said. "Now, show me where the blood was coming from."

"No, no need," she said flatly. "I'm fine now. Go do whatever it is you were doing when I called you in here. Really, I'm fine. Go on."

When Jane emerged from the bathroom an hour later, she still wouldn't answer any of my questions. No matter how much I pleaded, she refused to be seen by a doctor and angrily told me never to ask her again. She went about her usual Saturday activities as if nothing had happened.

I was shaken. Did she really have cancer? How could she be sure unless she let a doctor look at it? She might be right...but she might be wrong. How could she possibly know how serious it was? When she told me that she was "dying," did she say that because of the bleeding, or did she know more than she was letting on?

Everything about her medical condition was unclear. But what was abundantly clear was her desire not to discuss it. I had to decide: do I use whatever limited leverage I might have to keep confronting her, or do I comply with her wishes by denying that any of this ever happened?

I chose the latter. I spoke to no one.

* * *

Now, I had to confront the fact that yesterday, the day of her pulmonary embolus, and for many, many days before that, I had known about Jane's breast cancer. I had never seen it and I had no idea how serious or widespread it was, but I could no longer tell myself that I'd been unaware of it.

Jane's revelation on the bathroom floor made me realize that some of her inexplicable behaviors—many involving a ratcheting down of intimacy and communication, and a ratcheting up of compulsive tics—had arisen from the anxiety she must have felt after first discovering her cancer. Those changes had begun six years before the bathroom floor incident, which meant that, by the time of her pulmonary embolus, Jane had been hiding her cancer for a decade. And I had been deeply complicit in her secrecy for the last four years.

Why had I acquiesced? In part, it was just another example of giving Jane whatever space and support she needed to calm her anxieties. My habit of accommodating her eccentricities had become deeply ingrained.

But there was more. On that Saturday afternoon four years before her collapse, I had witnessed a medical emergency—the bleeding—and learned about my wife's shocking cancer diagnosis. I'd had an overwhelming impulse to act but suppressed it because Jane commanded me to, and I felt powerless to oppose her. What was that about?

There was no better feeling in the world than being in Jane's good graces. Her formidable intelligence and finely honed tastes combined to make her approval something special. A nod made you feel like a million bucks. And for exactly the same reasons, her disfavor was crushing. This was true for anyone who interacted with Jane but, of course, I felt it much more intensely because love was added to the mix.

I had crossed Jane once or twice in our marriage and her response had been to withdraw—not just her affection but everything. Being frozen out felt like the worst punishment imaginable. I would respond with a desperate scramble to find anything that might restore me to her favor, including, in this case, a promise not to do anything about her breast cancer.

Now I felt deeply ashamed of my inaction. Fear of Jane's displeasure was an absurd excuse. I asked myself, what kind of husband could stand by idly for four years while his wife's breast cancer grew? I'm still asking that question.

SIX

I brought Jane's iPod with me when I returned to the ICU the next morning, the start of her second full day in intensive care. Back when she still traveled for work, Jane used to invent strategies to mitigate the misery of being away from home. Her favorite was to distract herself with music. Knowing her tastes, I'd made her a playlist of songs from the 1960s and '70s. One of the things I loved about Jane was that, like me, she knew the lyrics of every Beatles song, so they were well represented along with lots of Elvis Costello, of course.

On travel days, Jane would nervously scan the street in front of our apartment, looking for her taxi to the airport. As soon as it arrived, she would grab her iPod and pop in the earbuds. She'd hit play when she got into the cab and would keep the music going while she passed through security and boarded her plane. She wouldn't take the earbuds out until she was safely in her hotel room. She did the same thing on her way home. I can still see her walking through the front door, earbuds in place, pulling her suitcase behind her.

The first thing I did that morning in the ICU, after telling Jane that I loved her, was to put the earbuds in her ears and start the playlist. I thought that maybe she'd dream that she was stuck in a middle seat on the worst flight ever.

I had a hard time reconciling my intent with the inert body in the hospital bed. Her face was so disconcertingly impassive—eyelids shut, corners of her mouth turned down around her breathing tube. The effect was off-putting, as if she were telling us all to leave her alone.

This was so different from the alert, engaged, and active Jane everyone knew. One of her most appealing characteristics was that, when she spoke to you, you had her undivided attention. Her clear blue eyes would bore into yours as she carefully weighed whatever it was you were saying.

Given the intensity of her focus, most people would not have called her a fidgeter. But she was. World class. Usually, Jane's interlocutors were so intent on marshalling their responses to her well-crafted and logically impenetrable arguments that they didn't notice how her jaw was in constant motion as she worked her chewing gum. Or how, while she chewed, she twirled the ends of her long hair around two fingers of her right hand, first one way then the other, never pausing. Some part of her was always in constant, restless motion.

Not now, of course. The blood clot, the Propofol, and god knows what else had rendered her immobile. She was nearly unrecognizable without her open eyes, sharp tongue, and fidgets.

* * *

I stayed with Jane all that day and into the early evening. As I was getting ready to go home, I looked up and saw Eric walk into the room. He had come straight from the airport.

This was a grand and compassionate gesture, but it unsettled me—I was whipsawed between opposing thoughts. On one hand, I was reassured that a trusted colleague would now be caring for Jane and even a little relieved that I would be sharing Jane's secret with someone. On the other hand, I felt exposed and angry. Eric would see the mass on Jane's chest and would draw inferences about our lives together. He would conclude, accurately, that marital intimacy had been replaced by years of deception. He had no right to know that much about Jane and me—but I had no choice.

Although I had warned Eric that Jane was intubated, the reality seemed to take him by surprise and he asked me lots of questions about how much damage her heart and lungs had sustained. It was as if Jane's breast cancer had been an incidental discovery, a sideshow to the main event of her pulmonary embolism. I suggested that he refocus and take a look at the cancer.

Eric pulled down Jane's johnnie and gently undid some of Sue's bandages. I didn't know what he was expecting, but it sure wasn't this. I gave him lots of credit for not losing his composure.

"Well, this does look pretty bad," he said, "but we'll figure something out. There's nothing we need to do about the breast cancer now. We can come up with a plan after she's out of the ICU. Meanwhile, how are *you* doing?"

I wasn't ready to bare my soul to Eric or anybody else. I told him that I was okay, all things considered, and that I deeply appreciated his willingness to take care of Jane. I told him there was no way I could ever repay him.

"But," I said for what felt like the millionth time, "there's one very important thing. Please don't tell anyone about Jane's breast cancer; she wouldn't want anyone at the Farber to know about it. People will hear about the cancer eventually, but I want to let Jane control the narrative as much as possible."

So, there it was yet again. A frank admission of secrecy and weirdness in our relationship. But Eric took it in stride and told me not to worry. He gave me a look that combined compassion, pity, bewilderment, and concern. He said he'd be back the next day. After he left, I sat with Jane for a few more minutes and then left to meet my daughter.

* * *

From the very start of our relationship, Jane made it clear that she did not want to have children. Ostensibly, she didn't want a child to disrupt her career plans. But I also think that the idea of being

51

responsible for another person's life scared her. I saw evidence of this in her decision to stop taking care of patients once she'd established herself on Dana Farber's faculty. She loved interacting with the people she cared for in the clinic but was petrified that she'd do something wrong that might harm them.

Whatever the reason, I accepted Jane's decision not to have children without argument because, after all, I had Anna. I figured that we'd simply incorporate Anna into our lives—she would become our daughter.

That was not to be. Signs of Jane's disinclination appeared soon after we started dating. Anna lived with her mother but, like most divorced dads who don't have custody, I tried to spend as much time as I could with her. Of course, my work schedule was unforgiving, which made weekends when I wasn't on call particularly precious. One Saturday during the first summer that Jane and I were together, I told her that I was planning to take Anna to the beach and that it would be wonderful if she'd join us. Jane was furious—she thought that weekends were for her and me alone. She barely spoke to me for the next two days.

I didn't know it then but this was the beginning of thirty years of "It's her or me" negotiations. From that point on, Jane would regularly berate me for having had a family before we met, saying, "I waited, why didn't you?" Her message seemed to be that our lives together were a kind of zero-sum affair in which my having had a child with someone else precluded her having one with me. I am embarrassed to say that it took me years to realize that Jane's irrationality and anger were rooted in her jealousy of Anna.

I also hate to admit that, far too often, I chose to keep Jane happy by not spending more time with my daughter. I deeply regret my inability to convince Jane that the choice she presented was a false one and that there would have been plenty of love to go around if we had integrated Anna into our lives. But we did not, and I am disappointed in myself for not forcing the issue.

Despite the strictures Jane had imposed, Anna and I maintained a bond. This was partly because of my eagerness to involve her in all the things Jane wouldn't do—concerts, Red Sox games, visiting my mother. Jane's absence gave me complete, unselfconscious freedom to be a father in those settings. I commiserated with Anna about school, about her stepsiblings, and, later, about boyfriends. I could be a sounding board when she tried on new identities. (As a teenager, Anna decided to become a vegetarian. When I asked her why, she replied that she lived in a small town and had a lot of time on her hands. She had a well-developed sense of humor.)

In contrast, Jane's disengagement was complete. She was utterly uninterested in joining Anna and me in these activities. She even refused to meet Anna's mother until I dragged her, mentally kicking and screaming, to Anna's high school graduation. Anna would have liked to see Jane be part of our lives together, but her absence did not prevent us from forging our own special relationship.

At the time of Jane's collapse, Anna was thirty-three, married, and the mother of an angelic boy—my grandson. He'd had some medical problems when he was born but was now doing well, thanks, in large part, to the attention and care he received from Anna and her husband. Jane's attitude had even melted a little after the grandchild appeared. She could be bestirred every so often to join me when I checked in with Anna's family who lived a few minutes away.

I had called Anna from the ICU that morning to let her know that Jane was in the hospital and asked if she'd have dinner with me. Despite my last-minute invitation, she left her husband and son to fend for themselves and agreed to meet me at a local restaurant. She was already there when I walked in.

I was always a little shocked whenever I saw the adult Anna. *Who is this gorgeous person? Is she really the grown-up version of my little girl?* Anna had become a real beauty—tall, athletic, high cheekbones under radiant eyes, a thousand-watt smile, all framed by long, flowing brown hair. She had my coloring and some of my features—my friends said she looked like I would if I were good looking.

As soon as Anna saw me, she gave me a long hug.

"Oh, Daddy," she said. "I'm so sorry about all of this."

"Thank you, sweetheart," I said. "It means a lot that you'd have dinner with me."

"Are you kidding?" she said as we sat down. "I'd do anything for you. Tell me what happened."

I told her the story: Jane's collapse at work, the pulmonary embolus, and the discovery of her advanced breast cancer. I spared her the gory details about the tumor itself and elided the business about Jane hiding her cancer from everyone.

"I don't think I've ever heard something so terrible," Anna said. "How are you holding up?"

"I suppose I'm doing as well as I can be, given the circumstances," I replied.

I kept waiting for Anna to catch the inconsistency at the heart of the story—the sudden discovery of advanced breast cancer in a medically sophisticated woman—and start asking uncomfortable questions. But she didn't. Maybe she was too shocked to notice. Or maybe she did notice but thought this wouldn't be the right time to probe.

"Please, please," she said, "if there's anything Ted or I can do to help, you have to let us know."

"Thanks so much, sweetie," I said, "but there's really nothing that anyone can do now. I just have to keep hoping that she's got enough stamina, enough physical reserves to survive this. But I don't know, she might not."

Tears welled in Anna's eyes.

"Oh, Dad," she said, reaching for my arm. "Jane's in a great hospital being taken care of by great doctors. They'll pull her through."

"Thanks, Anna," I said. "You're a brick."

She was. Not just because she was being so supportive but because I was being so unfair. I had spent decades acceding to Jane's wishes not to incorporate Anna into our world. She had to have felt the sting of the rejection that I hadn't done nearly enough to counteract. Now, at the first sign of serious trouble, here I was turning to my daughter for support. She had every right to be respectful but cool—to keep me at the same distance I had kept her. I would have deserved it. Instead, Anna sat with me, talked with me, and cried with me. Her empathy was boundless. She had figured out a way to buoy my spirits while acknowledging the gravity of the situation and without resorting to trite and empty reassurances.

What a relief that our relationship had survived. Still, because I hadn't stood up to Jane, I had deprived Anna of any semblance of a normal family life with a father and stepmother. That's my fault, and although I'll spend the rest of my life trying to make amends, there won't be enough time.

* * *

As I walked home to my empty apartment after dinner, I started ticking through the people I still needed to call to let them know about Jane. There was my sister who lived with her second husband a few hours away in Vermont. She'd get what was going on. Her first husband had died of cancer soon after they were married. He was older than my sister but was far too young when he died.

That would do it for family. But there were others I absolutely had to call, starting with Michael and Christopher, our closest friends. Michael had been an oncology fellow with Jane at Dana-Farber and the two had made an instant connection. He and his partner, Christopher, were the only people who Jane had let into our bubble. They had moved away ten years earlier but we had maintained our friendship. They would want to know what had happened.

I also needed to talk to Deb, an oncologist in the Division of Population Sciences that Jane led at Dana-Farber. Hospitals are gossip mills, and it was likely that Deb had already heard about Jane's collapse and that she was in the ICU. But, since she would likely be the acting head of the division in Jane's absence, she would need to know a few details in order to understand when—and if—Jane would be coming back to work. I could tell Deb enough to help inform her planning without revealing the secrets that Jane wouldn't want her to know.

That would be enough. Just thinking about the calls I'd have to make tomorrow made me feel exhausted. I went straight to bed when I got home.

SEVEN

The next seventy-two hours were a blur. Little distinguished one day from the next other than the agonizingly slow improvement in Jane's condition. I lived for the better numbers on her monitors. By her fourth day in the ICU, the team was so encouraged by her progress that they started to taper her sedatives. Although this didn't bring her to full consciousness, it did have the unfortunate effect of waking her up just enough to make her aware that she was uncomfortable. She began to pull at her breathing tube and her intravenous lines. So, later in the day, when I returned to the ICU after running some errands, I was dismayed by the sight of my wife in restraints—her wrists were tied to the bedrails. That broke my heart. While restraints are often used for intubated patients, they are also for patients who are demented and unable to follow commands. That was how I'd used them when I was in training. I couldn't imagine anything sadder than my brilliant wife being tied up like a patient with Alzheimer's.

Still, the ICU team thought Jane was doing well enough to start the process of weaning her from the ventilator. This was a delicate dance that involved lightening her sedation bit by bit and turning off the ventilator—with the tube still in her throat—to see if she could breathe on her own. The first few times they tried it, Jane's blood pressure shot up to dangerous levels and her lung function deteriorated so badly that the ventilator had to be turned back on. The team was frustrated. They thought she was ready to breathe without assistance, but apparently, she wasn't.

I was frustrated too. Everything else seemed to be moving in the right direction and I was desperate to see the breathing tube removed so that I could talk to her. I was sitting next to Jane's bed, obsessing about her medical condition, when I had a random thought.

Jane was a smoker when we first met. She had started in college, as had I, so the smoke itself didn't bother me. What did bother me was the fact that, in every room in her apartment, there were ash-trays overflowing with butts. I never figured out what would finally motivate her to empty them but it only happened rarely. Jane also smoked in bed, and I inferred that she had been doing so for years because her sheets were riddled with cigarette holes.

Jane continued to smoke all through her residency, often joining the nurses in their offices or in the stairwell to share a cigarette. But she knew that she would have to quit before starting her oncology fellowship—smoking would not be tolerated at a cancer hospital. So, one Saturday in May, just before her fellowship started, I bought a box of nicotine gum; Nicorette was the brand name. I put it and Jane in the passenger seat of our little Honda Civic and headed west. I drove on secondary roads for hours while Jane cold-tur-keyed. We meandered all the way to the little town of Florence in western Massachusetts, where I had something to eat at the Miss Florence Diner. Jane didn't have an appetite. Then we slowly drove home the way we came.

Jane never had another cigarette, but she also never stopped chewing Nicorette. That gum was her constant companion for the next twenty-five years. Each piece came in a clear plastic case that she called a "house." Whenever she took a fresh piece of gum out of its house, she would replace it with the one she had been chewing. For some reason, though, she could not be bothered to throw out the house with the used gum. For years, she would accumulate a mound of plastic houses filled with chewed Nicorette next to her desktop computer at home—it would grow to several inches in height—until something clicked and she decided to toss them. The nicotine gum houses got exactly the same treatment that her cigarette butts used to get.

Now, in the ICU, it occurred to me that Jane had not had any Nicorette since her collapse. She had been chewing that stuff daily for decades—maybe she was in nicotine withdrawal.

Or maybe this was just a dumb idea. Back when I was taking care of patients, I'd listen to well-meaning family members offer suggestions about how the hospital team could better care for their loved ones. Most doctors are sufficiently courteous not to roll their eyes, but, often enough, they'll dismiss these ideas with patronizing smiles. In this case, of course, I was a doctor myself but my long absence from the world of patient care was likely to make my medical notions more dangerous than helpful. So, I was self-conscious about offering up my opinions. I didn't want to be one of "those" husbands.

Despite my misgivings, the next time the ICU team rounded on Jane, I tamped down my embarrassment and sheepishly floated my Nicorette idea. To my surprise, they took me seriously. I don't know if they really thought there was any merit to the suggestion or if they were just indulging me, but they ordered up some nicotine patches and put one on Jane's arm. The next time they tried to wean her from the ventilator, she did much better. Her blood pressure remained stable and she was able to take several breaths on her own. That was progress.

The problem now was that Jane was awake. She was acutely aware of the breathing tube in her airway and realized that she couldn't talk. She tugged at her restraints. Her eyes darted wildly around the room, communicating her distress. I tried to calm her by putting my face directly in front of hers and repeating the things I had said to her when she was unconscious: you've had a large pulmonary embolus and you're on a ventilator in the ICU at the Brigham. Her eyes widened in what I interpreted as terror and disbelief. I told her that I loved her and that she was getting better—her eyes seemed to soften a little—and that the team was giving her a trial of breathing without the help of the vent. But then her oxygen levels started declining, so they increased her sedation and turned the machine back on.

They spent the rest of that day attempting to get Jane to breathe on her own. I tried to be there each time the team lightened her sedation so that I could talk to her, comfort her, and encourage her to breathe. Unfortunately, every time they pushed that boulder up the hill, it rolled right back down. By the next day, though, Jane was a little stronger and better able to maintain her oxygen levels during the challenges. When the team finally decided that she didn't need the ventilator anymore, they pulled the tube from her throat.

Seeing Jane extubated was one of the most moving experiences of my life. It was as if she had come back from the dead. I hugged her and kissed her and told her that I loved her.

Jane looked at me without saying anything. All week long, I had been suppressing the fear that Jane might have suffered brain damage. That kind of thing can occur when someone's oxygen levels plummet during a major collapse like the one she had. Is that why she's looking at me so blankly? Does she even know who I am?

"Are you okay, hon?" I asked.

"Yeah, I think so," she said and smiled. She recognized me.

Jane was awake and talking. For nearly a week, I'd been nervously hoping this moment would arrive. Hoping, of course, because being freed from the ventilator meant that Jane would have survived and our life together wasn't over. Nervous because now we would need to talk about her secrets and the havoc they had caused.

But, as it happened, that difficult discussion would have to wait. Even though Jane knew who I was and could hold up her end of a conversation, she was not herself. Most striking was her lack of concern about the trauma she had just lived through. She asked me a few times to tell her about what had happened, and I dutifully repeated the story of her pulmonary embolus, her collapse, and how she had been intubated in the ICU. In response to each successive horror, she looked at me with a half-smile and said, "Uh-huh." I wasn't sure what to make of her attitude, but it felt weird.

There was more. During one of our conversations, Jane glanced over my shoulder and nonchalantly asked if I could see the rats climbing up the curtain over her doorway. That was certainly disturbing. I went to the door and ran my hand over the curtain. I told Jane that there were no rats and that she was seeing things. Jane insisted, with a smile, that they were really there. Great. She hadn't lost her stubbornness.

Later, when the ICU team made its rounds, I told them about the rats. They seemed unconcerned and said that these kinds of hallucinations were common in patients in the ICU. So later, after they left, when Jane asked, "Umm...I don't suppose you see the river of blood pouring down the wall, do you?" I was somewhat less worried. But it was still unsettling.

Jane's lack of concern about these frightening visions was impressive. She would mention them in passing and patiently listen as I told her that they weren't real. Even when she disagreed and insisted that the rats and the blood were actually there, she was completely calm. In some ways, this behavior felt like an adaptive response to her circumstances: her medical condition had been dire and her stay in the ICU frightening. I learned later that it can also be a component of the post-traumatic stress disorder that many patients suffer after being in the ICU. If this blasé attitude kept her anxiety and stress at bay, I was all for it. But I hoped it would go away soon. I wanted the old Jane back.

Now that Jane was off the ventilator, she could be moved out of the ICU. She was transferred to a huge private room that had a daybed so I could sleep there. There was also a television on the wall, which she wouldn't let me turn off at night.

As her condition improved, she stopped hallucinating—that was a relief. But her visions were replaced by a new behavior that was nearly as disturbing. Jane began to insist that she knew exactly what I was about to say or do before I said or did it. She had enough insight to admit that this intense feeling of déjà vu was unusual, but she was adamant that it was real.

I had been sitting next to her bed, reading a magazine, when she told me about her new superpower for the third time that morning. I thought that some gentle reality testing might be in order.

"Hon, I'm going to read a few sentences in this article," I said. "You tell me what comes next and then we'll see if you're right. Okay?"

She agreed. I read two paragraphs aloud and then stopped.

"What's next?" I asked.

"I don't know," Jane replied casually.

I read the next three sentences, at which point Jane interrupted me with a shout.

"I *knew* that's what would be next!"

I didn't argue. Reality testing can only take you so far.

But I was worried: what if this stuff didn't improve? Jane's brain was her proudest asset and the way her mind worked was one of the things I loved most about her. It would be devastating if she were permanently incapacitated by these delusions. Many years earlier, my mother had had a massive heart attack and, like Jane, was placed on a ventilator. She, too, woke up after a long ICU stay but was never the same. My experience with my mother was tilting me toward pessimism, but I couldn't help it. The fact that Jane's delusions weren't bothering her was a blessing for her, but it only made things sadder for me. I couldn't believe how much had changed in such a short time.

EIGHT

The specter of brain damage would be horrifying for anyone, but it was particularly so for Jane. She was whip-smart, maybe the smartest person I'd ever met, and a great talker. Being older than her peers, she surveyed the medical world with a gimlet eye that made her seem sophisticated even when she wasn't.

Admittedly, her intelligence came with an edge. Jane was intensely competitive: Scrabble was a duel to the death and Monopoly was a blood sport. She had a deep-seated need to win every argument, although her merciless eviscerations were often couched in folksy vernacular that could catch you off guard. A disagreement might begin with her saying, "Liar, liar, pants on fire," followed by a devastatingly logical takedown. She might then take her victory lap by saying, "So, there, Mister Smarty-Pantsy!"

Jane was a reader, having either inherited or adopted her father's passion for language and books. But not all books. She thought modernism was crap and wasn't shy about eloquently belittling me if I had the temerity to say that I liked Joyce or Proust. She preferred American Realists like Dreiser and Norris.

She was intensely analytical, with an uncanny ability to identify the critically important components of a problem, discard the irrelevant ones, and dispassionately weigh all of the facts before coming to a conclusion. Her tough-mindedness often led to unpopular positions, especially in the world of clinical research, where she was an early advocate for mitigating conflicts of interest. While all scientists need to be rigorously objective in their work, the stakes are higher for clinical scientists because their research involves human beings. If a patient were to suffer a serious side effect from the experimental treatment being tested, the clinical trialist must be prepared to remove the patient from the trial or even shut it down altogether. Nothing but the patient's well-being can influence that decision, just as nothing but a clear-eyed assessment of the trial data can determine whether it was "successful," the label trialists use when the experimental drug is effective. (It could be argued that a clear demonstration of a drug's ineffectiveness is also a "successful" trial, but that's not how the term of art is used.)

Like others, Jane believed that an investigator's financial interest in the success of a trial could compromise their objectivity. For example, if the physician owned stock in the pharmaceutical company that developed the study drug, a successful trial would raise share prices and, therefore, the value of the physician's portfolio. Or the physician might have a lucrative consulting arrangement with the company, which would be sustained or even enhanced by a positive trial outcome.

Although many doctors believe that their objectivity could not possibly be compromised by outside considerations like these, Jane was familiar with studies that documented the untoward influence of even trivial amounts of money on a doctor's judgment. A sufficient consensus had formed around the effects of financial interests so that rules had begun to appear that restricted the participation of anyone with such interests in clinical research.

But Jane pressed the logic of her position to its conclusion, one that some considered extreme. She insisted that the lure of fame and professional advancement had the potential to influence academic physicians every bit as much as money in their pockets—that an investigator's judgment could be affected by the reputational enhancement they'd enjoy if the clinical trial they were running were to have a successful outcome. The only way to counter this insidious effect, according to Jane, would be to prohibit anyone who had conceived of or designed a trial from having anything to do with its execution. She suggested that the Farber hire a cadre of physicians whose job would be to run the clinical trials developed by others. They'd be insulated from the career-enhancing influence of a positive trial because their performance evaluations would be based on how skillfully they ran the trials, not on the trials' results.

This idea was anathema to the Farber's faculty who wanted to run the trials that tested their own ideas, so it never gained traction. But she was right, and she had reached her conclusion through a dispassionate analysis of the facts.

Jane tried to employ this skill in her own life. For the most part, she would use her cool-headed analyses to inform choices she needed to make about her professional career and did so to great effect. Sometimes, though, logic deserted her and momentous decisions could be rooted in emotion.

"You know," she said at one of our Friday dinners soon after she'd joined the faculty, "I don't think I want to take care of patients anymore."

"Really?" I said, a little surprised. "You're so good at it."

"What do you mean?" she asked.

"I mean that everyone who's ever seen you in a clinical setting—patients, nurses, other doctors—think that you're a fantastic clinician."

"I suppose," she said, half-heartedly.

"And your patients love you," I continued. "Look at all the gifts they bring when they come for their appointments. Your office is filled with them. Even the patients who've died, their families send these long letters to the Farber talking about how you were such a kind and caring doctor."

"I suppose," she said again, a little quieter this time.

"And you were chief resident at the Brigham, for Christ's sake!" I was going to add that being chief was an honor I was never offered, but I didn't.

"Means nothing," she said.

I paused to see what she'd say next.

"*You're* not seeing patients anymore," she said. "Why's that okay for you?"

"I figured out that I can't do two things at once and do them both well," I said. "I had to make a choice and I chose research. Look, I don't think there's anything wrong if you decide to do that too. I just think you're actually capable of doing both. I don't want you to sell yourself short if you like doing clinical medicine."

"I liked my patients, but I never liked clinical medicine," she said emphatically. "There's a difference."

"I get that," I said. "But why don't you like it?"

"Because all we do in oncology is make people miserable," she said. "I cannot spend my professional life signing medication orders that make helpless people throw up, lose their hair, bleed out, or die from infections. They're already sick enough."

That was the nub. Jane was terrified of hurting people—a fear that was rooted in her deep empathy for suffering patients and a worry that she might inadvertently make things worse. So, it was a tremendous relief for Jane that, by focusing on research, she could fashion a successful life in medicine that did not involve worrying about patients.

But what kind of research would she do? Choosing a scientific focus is a momentous, high-stakes decision. Choices made at this early juncture can determine so much of what happens later in a career—success or failure, professional advancement or stasis, happiness or misery. I had been in an MD/PhD program in medical school and learned how to use molecular biology to understand disease, so it was no surprise that I wanted to continue that kind of research. In fact, when I started my own laboratory, the genetic revolution was in full swing and most of the young faculty in my cohort were eager to work on the molecular basis of cancer.

Jane took a very different tack. As a fellow, she had been trained to treat cancer with the tools at hand, mainly chemotherapy drugs. But she questioned whether the severe toxicities they caused—the very ones that made her shy away from clinical oncology—were too high a price to pay for the few extra months of life they generally bought. So, she created a new field: the science of outcomes measurement in oncology. She attracted like-minded colleagues and together they developed methods for determining whether cancer treatments produce improvements in meaningful outcomes like the quality of someone's life, not just its length. Jane asked whether patients who are given all the facts about chemotherapy—what it could do and, especially, could not do—would want to be treated at all. She discovered that many people suffering from the most common cancers would rather die peacefully at home than undergo the tortures of chemotherapy. This, too, made her unpopular in some oncology circles, but it made her famous.

Jane's career took off like a rocket. She and her team made advances in integrating patient preferences into treatment plans, documenting the futility of ineffective treatment, and optimizing governmental health policy to improve the lives of whole populations. She also made important contributions to the way we think about end-of-life care in cancer, emphasizing the importance of providing comfort and palliation over administering marginally effective and toxic treatments.

To manage all this work, Jane created a Center for Outcomes and Policy Research at Dana-Farber, which drew international attention. She won lots of awards and, in short order, was appointed chief of the Division of Population Sciences at Dana-Farber. Around the same time, she became one of the small number of women to be granted tenure as a professor at Harvard Medical School.

* * *

Jane had fashioned a successful academic career for herself—no mean feat for a woman at Harvard. But she'd done something else. I've never seen anyone else who could inspire such fierce loyalty in the people who worked in her field and, particularly, in those who she'd trained. And it wasn't just loyalty. Jane became a beloved figure and role model who inspired an "I'd take a bullet for that woman" level of devotion.

Why?

I'd asked myself that question a few times over the past twenty years and I found myself asking it again when I came home after another day of sitting with Jane in the hospital. The question had become particularly pointed because I had just started to allow myself to be angry. In fact, while making dinner for myself that night, I realized that I was thoroughly pissed about how Jane had put me in such an impossible position. I had lied to her family—would they ever trust me again?—and I was urging her doctors to hide a fundamentally unhideable illness from her colleagues. When the truth finally emerged, I was going to feel embarrassed and decidedly idiotic.

I was still fuming when I sat down at my desk after dinner to deal with the email backlog I'd been avoiding. Waiting in my inbox were over two hundred unopened messages. Word had gotten out about Jane's collapse, and her colleagues had written to me with their expressions of shock, concern, and support.

As I scrolled through the messages, I couldn't help being struck by their tone—they all talked about how amazing, talented, and wonderful Jane was—and the way they contrasted with my own angry thoughts. I'd been ruminating about Jane's unacceptable behaviors and the horrible consequences they'd wrought, but here were messages from literally hundreds of people who felt compelled to write about her virtues. The hero worship was on full display.

I sat back and asked myself again, *Why? Where did this come from?*

I'm sure that it had something to do with the electric thrill people felt when Jane focused her attention on them. She could make the targets of her interest believe that they were the most important human beings who'd ever lived and that she'd be willing to do anything to help them. It was the talent of a skilled politician but without the insincerity. And while I might have expected this kind of seduction to work on trainees whose careers could benefit from her mentorship, I saw the same admiration and devotion in colleagues up and down the academic hierarchy.

At the top, among tenured professors and department chairs, Jane had a very specific following. The kind of research she did—inferring cancer-related outcomes from massive datasets—required the use of complex statistical methods. Because she understood the power of those methods, Jane had tremendous respect for the mathematicians and statisticians who had developed them. Growing up, Jane herself had been a nerd—a pale, skinny kid with thick cat-eye glasses, always tall for her age, and way smarter than her peers. She maintained a nerd's appreciation for her own kind even after her transformation into a swan who wore contacts.

To understand the loyalty she inspired from this crowd, you have to imagine the setting. A bunch of math geeks who'd spent their lives surrounded by other math geeks suddenly find themselves working with an elegant creature who doesn't just tolerate them— she actually likes them. Jane told me about one of her colleagues, a preeminent scientist who, having heard from Jane about her love for *The Simpsons*, idly wondered whether, because the characters have only four fingers on each hand, they lived in a base-eight world. Jane thought that was hilarious. No doubt he'd been making jokes like this since he was a teenager, but I'll bet this was the first time one of the cool kids had laughed. No wonder he and his ilk loved her.

Then there were her trainees. Ambitious youngsters are desperately hungry for attention from their accomplished elders. They don't yet know the ropes and are forever worried that they're making the wrong decisions. Jane loved working with the up-and-coming, and they loved working with her. When she turned her attention to them, offering advice largely drawn from her own experiences, her personal touch made them feel special.

In a way, though, this was a feint. Jane was an intensely private person. In the right setting, she could be gregarious and regale listeners with stories about herself that were entertaining and very funny, but they tended to be superficial. They were usually about "things that happened"—either to her or near her—all told in a way that revealed very little. Occasionally, she might lift a corner of the veil, especially when talking to trainees or junior faculty she was fond of. These young professionals felt like they had been given a special gift—a privileged glimpse of Jane's interior world that made them even more devoted to her. But the truth was that she hadn't told them anything about her private self.

Among her first trainees was Deb, a brilliant and precocious young doctor who already had inklings about how she might develop a successful academic career. What Jane provided were the tools and confidence to think even bigger. Academic preeminence comes to those who publish scholarly papers in a handful of top-tier journals like *The New England Journal of Medicine*. Because competition for limited editorial space is so fierce, articles that merely describe excellent science won't make the cut. Jane had a canny sense about ways to frame a paper's "story" so that editors would feel compelled to accept it. This is what she did for Deb—by helping her craft work that found a home in high-profile journals, it catapulted Deb's career.

Later, when Deb moved to New York, Jane continued to watch over her, providing advice and sponsoring her for memberships on important committees that raised her professional profile. She worked hard to bring Deb back to the Farber a decade later and anoint her as the eventual successor to lead her division.

But Jane's relationships with her trainees were not always smooth. She could not be relied upon to rein in her critical tendencies and would occasionally lace her guidance with withering criticism. Working with Jane was like playing with fire. In supportive mode, she was attractive, seductive, and mesmerizing. But you could get burned.

Before Deb left for New York, she discovered that she was finally pregnant after years of struggling with infertility. Unfortunately, the blessed event interfered with Jane's timeline for completing a high-profile research paper Deb had been working on.

"So," Jane asked her shortly before the due date, "how much maternity leave do you plan on taking?"

"Six weeks, I guess," said Deb. (This was before policies defining leave were well established.)

"Oh," said Jane. "Okay." She paused, tilting her head to one side and twisting her hair.

"You know," Jane continued, looking at Deb, "it's interesting to think about the professional women we've known who've had kids."

"What do you mean?" asked Deb.

"Well, take Caryn, for example. She returned to work full-time a few days after giving birth. Or Peg. Remember when she had herself wheeled over here to run a meeting right after she delivered? She still had an IV in her arm." Jane chuckled.

"And, of course," she continued, "there was Jill, who also somehow didn't miss a beat."

"Yes, sure," said Deb. "I know all of them."

"I just find it interesting," Jane continued with mock thoughtfulness, "that there seems to be an inverse correlation between the amount of time some women spend at home after giving birth and their degree of academic success."

Devastating words to hear from your mentor. Deb once told me that some of the meanest things anyone ever said to her had come out of Jane's mouth. But she still loved her and, to Deb's credit, she took her six weeks of maternity leave and still managed to be successful.

Now, back at Dana-Farber, Deb was still devoted to Jane. After I'd spoken to her about Jane's condition, Deb had come to the ICU a few times to provide support for me but also to see Jane. I wouldn't let her. After Jane's transfer to a regular hospital room, she tried again.

"You know I wouldn't dream of bothering her," Deb said. "But we all love Jane and, knowing her, I think she'd want to hear that everything is still functioning smoothly in her division."

"It's great that you care for her so much," I said. "It's really lovely. But she's not ready to see anyone."

"Sure, sure," Deb said quickly. "I get it. It's just that we're all so worried about her. And worried about you too. I only want to be helpful. Make sense?"

"Yes, and thank you," I said. "I just think that, right now, Jane's still too unstable to be able to appreciate a visit."

I was finessing the main point—Jane's breast cancer. I assumed that the critical information had not yet been leaked. I also assumed that if Deb saw Jane, she might ask questions along the lines of "Why did this happen?" and I couldn't allow that yet.

"Okay, of course," she said. "Meanwhile, though, let me know what I can do for you. I can bring over some dinners. It's no work for me and it would give you one less thing to worry about."

"What a generous offer," I said. "Thanks so much. But I'll be staying at the hospital for the duration and having my meals here. I really do appreciate the kindness, though."

The charade would have to end at some point but not just yet.

NINE

I spent the next seven days and nights at the hospital. Jane's room was on an upper floor with an enormous window that looked out on a park. Our pastoral view was soon obstructed by a mountain of bouquets and orchids that piled up on the sill and grew larger each day. Everyone from hospital presidents to family members sent flowers. It was as if the medical community had been holding its breath while Jane was in the ICU and was collectively exhaling now that it knew she had survived.

Jane slowly got stronger and her thinking became clearer. Dietitians advanced her to solid food, and physical therapists got her out of bed. Her brief, vertical excursions at the bedside were dicey. She could barely stand, and it was clear that she was struggling to do even the simplest things on her own.

I had known from the start that if Jane survived her ordeal, I would be caring for her at home, but I hadn't allowed myself to consider the prospect in any practical way. When she was in the ICU and it looked like she might die, I avoided imagining her back in our apartment fearing I might jinx the outcome. Then, as her condition improved, I still avoided thinking about it because the very idea of being responsible for Jane at home was terrifying.

But, whether I was ready or not, Jane had improved enough for her doctors to think about sending her home. Hospital discharge planners met with me to discuss what would come next. One of them floated the idea of sending Jane to a rehabilitation hospital as an intermediate step before going home. I nixed that. After my mother's heart attack, my father took care of her at home. My mom had often said that she would rather die than go to a nursing home. So, my father arranged to keep her in her own home regardless of her physical or mental state and, before he died, he made my sister and me promise that we would do the same. We kept the promise and, years later, she died in her own bed.

This was the way my father, not a demonstrative man, showed his love for my mother. I'm sure that I had internalized this behavior and now applied it to Jane—a truly loving husband would find a way to keep his sick wife at home. Not surprisingly, this was Jane's preference too. She wanted to be in her own bed watching her own TV, and I promised her that I would figure out a way to make that happen.

What my promise actually entailed became clearer as representatives from various health services paraded through Jane's hospital room. I would need to set up daily visits with nurses from the hospital's home care department. I would have to hire aides who could help me move Jane and bathe her and stay overnight if necessary. I would have to rent a walker, a shower seat, and a bedside toilet. I would have to rent an oxygen generator, backup oxygen tanks, and yards of plastic tubing. I would have to buy a reclining chair for Jane to sit in so that she could spend time out of bed, and it would have to have a motor that could raise the seat to lift her to a standing position. I would have to buy a wheelchair so that I could get her around the apartment. Finally, I would have to arrange for an ambulance to take her home.

I tried to suppress my panic as I signed the dozens of forms needed to put this machinery in place. I was on my own—I had no friends or family to talk to about my decisions, and Jane was still blissfully unconcerned about her circumstances.

Discharge was scheduled for Saturday, two weeks and one day after her lunchtime collapse, but our apartment was in no shape to receive someone who would need around-the-clock medical care. So, on Friday afternoon, I left Jane in her hospital room and drove to Bed Bath & Beyond. My thinking wasn't particularly organized. I knew we needed things that were sold there but I didn't know exactly what, so I hadn't made a shopping list. I was hoping that I could just walk up and down the aisles and whatever we needed would catch my eye.

My strategy worked well enough. I saw a blue foam "egg crate" mattress cover and put it in my shopping cart. I knew that Jane would be spending most of her time in bed and thought that it might make her more comfortable and prevent bedsores. I tossed a couple of sheet sets into the cart along with four pillows and pillowcases. I saw a "sit-up" pillow with arms. That looked promising—Jane could use it while she had her meals in bed. Into the cart. A serving tray with short fold-down legs called to me—I could use it to bring her those meals. Ooh, an intercom—I could put one unit on Jane's bedside table and the other next to my bed in the guest room. That way she could call for me in the night if she needed anything. Finally, I saw a set of storage boxes that looked like they might fit in the top drawer of Jane's dresser. I could use them to hold scissors, gauze, tape, and other things we would need for bandaging her tumor. I gingerly placed the boxes atop the wobbly mountain of stuff in the shopping cart and made my way to the checkout counter.

I took everything home and carried the shopping bags into the bedroom of our condominium. It wasn't exactly a designer's dream, but sometimes—and this was one of those times—I'd look around and think about how far Jane and I had come. When we first started dating, I would spend just about every night at her place in Cambridge. That apartment was appalling. For one thing, it was completely overrun with cockroaches. They were everywhere—scuttling over every horizontal surface and crawling up the walls. Jane had grown so accustomed to the infestation that she only rarely tried to kill them. And when she was roused to do so, she simply reached out and crushed them with a bare hand. I shuddered each time she did that.

Every room in her apartment was a disaster in some way but the bedroom was hopeless. Its tiny closet gave Jane an excuse to leave piles of clothes on her dresser, on a rundown chair in the corner, and on the floor. Its single window faced another building across a narrow courtyard so the shade was always pulled down tight. The overhead light was terrible so the room had a cave-like feel. And then, of course, there were the bedclothes riddled with cigarette burns.

The bedroom I was standing in now, thirty years later—bug-free with high ceilings and tenth-floor views through bay windows— couldn't have been more different.

Smiling at the memories of Jane's old place, I opened the shopping bags and started deploying my new purchases around the bedroom. I fitted the bed with its new accoutrements and put the extra sheets and pillowcases in the armoire. I placed one of the intercom units on the nightstand next to Jane's side of the bed and plugged it into the wall socket. Then, I turned to Jane's dresser. I opened the top drawer and began removing her underwear to make room for the new storage boxes I'd bought.

Suddenly, I was brought up short. At the back of the drawer, hidden behind her underwear, were dozens of prescription bottles. I stared at them, trying to figure out what I was looking at. I began reading the labels. Some were for antibiotics like the ones Jane used to prescribe for her bouts of abdominal pain. But these had all been recently filled, prescribed by Jane for herself over the past year. I'd known nothing about them.

I found more bottles—these held cancer drugs and Jane was again listed as the prescribing physician. It took me a minute to realize what this meant: Jane had been treating her cancer herself. I was stunned. A few of the prescriptions were for estrogen blockers but others were for toxic chemotherapy drugs. This was horrifying.

Jane, on her own initiative and without supervision, had been giving herself chemotherapy, risking life-threatening infections or bleeding.

I knew—as did Jane—that the most serious side effect of these drugs is their propensity to lower a patient's blood cell counts. If the number of white cells in the blood gets too low, patients can't fight infections. If the number of platelets in the blood gets too low, they can't clot when they bleed. Oncologists try to hold these disasters at bay by obtaining regular and frequent blood tests. If they see their patient's white cell or platelet numbers drifting downward, they decrease the dose of the chemotherapy drug to allow the patient's blood to recover.

Jane's secretive behavior would have kept her from asking anyone to check her blood counts because doing so would have meant revealing her diagnosis. Instead, she was flying blind. While I was trying to digest these dreadful facts, another part of my brain realized that her self-treatment explained some recent mysteries. During the past few years, I'd noticed that Jane would intermittently look paler than usual or she would take to her bed for a week. I now realized—the penny dropped with an almost audible thud—that Jane was experiencing the side effects of chemo as her blood counts reached their low point. I don't know how she managed not to kill herself.

While I was still reeling from my discovery, the doorbell rang. The technician from the oxygen company had arrived with the equipment I'd ordered. I gathered my wits and let him in. He wheeled the oxygen generator—an appliance about the size of a small refrigerator—into the bedroom. He showed me how to set it up and how to use the valves on the green backup tanks. I was disconcerted by his completely normal behavior—he seemed to think that this was just another routine delivery. Didn't he know that I'd just found out my wife was giving herself chemotherapy?

After the technician left, I grabbed a change of clothes and drove back to the hospital to spend Friday night with Jane. I said nothing about the pill bottles or the chemo—this was not the time. Of course, I'd been telling myself for decades that "this was not the time" whenever confrontations loomed with Jane, but this really wasn't the time.

While lying awake in Jane's hospital room that night, my insomnia driven by anticipatory dread of the next day's events, I replayed my pathetic thirty-year record of conflict avoidance. That gave me the privilege of watching the sun come up on Saturday morning, discharge day.

I got out of bed, checked on Jane—she was still asleep—and made a run to the cafeteria to get coffee and a bagel for my breakfast. I brought them back to Jane's room just as the discharge planners showed up. They were all over me to make sure that I hadn't forgotten anything. I hadn't. We'd be ready to go just as soon as I finished my breakfast, which I obligingly wolfed down.

Naturally, it wasn't until mid-afternoon that hospital transport came to get Jane out of bed and into a wheelchair. They took her to the hospital's main entrance where an oversized ambulance was waiting. It had a hydraulic platform that could accommodate a wheelchair—they called it a "chair car." The driver wheeled Jane onto the platform and secured her chair using an intricate system of heavy, woven cloth bands and locks. He raised the platform, slid it into the ambulance, and got into the driver's seat. I followed them in our car.

When we arrived at our apartment, the ambulance driver reversed the process and, just like that, there was Jane in a wheelchair at the back door of our building. The driver asked if we were okay and then took off before I could answer. I was scared to death but tried to radiate confidence as I asked Jane if she was excited to be home. She gave me a sidelong glance and said nothing.

I wheeled her into the elevator, still playing the self-assured spouse in control. I told her about the comfortable bed and her new sheets and how she could have anything she wanted for dinner. The home health aide was not scheduled to arrive for another few hours. I silently prayed that nothing bad would happen to Jane between now and then, and that I would be able to maintain my composure.

We got to our floor, and I clumsily maneuvered the wheelchair out of the elevator and into the narrow hallway leading to our front door. I unlocked it and wheeled my wife—my wife who had nearly died in the ICU, who had advanced breast cancer that she'd kept hidden, and who had been treating herself with chemo—into our apartment.

TEN

Jane's homecoming was a low-key affair. No banners, no cut flowers. I suppose I could have been a more enthusiastic one-man welcoming committee, but I couldn't afford any distractions—I was devoting all my attention to wheeling Jane into her bedroom without knocking over tables or scraping paint off walls. I managed to negotiate the ninety-degree turns in the narrow hallway that led to the bedroom—no barrier to the ambulatory—without inflicting too much damage and rolled the wheelchair into place next to Jane's bed. I was trying my best to project an aura of insouciant competence while suppressing the anxiety that was clamoring for my attention.

I locked the wheels and helped Jane stand. She gingerly put a hand on my shoulder to steady herself while I took off her coat and draped it over the back of the wheelchair. I slowly and methodically helped her out of her clothes, pausing now and then to give her a chance to catch her breath. I reached into the plastic bag the nurses had given us when we left the hospital and fished out one of the half-dozen johnnies they'd provided as parting gifts. I slipped it over Jane's arms, tied it loosely in the back, and eased her into bed. I activated the oxygen generator—it started making a quiet but annoying hum—and guided its plastic tubing over Jane's ears and under her nose so that the two small prongs at the end directed oxygen into her nostrils. I turned on the television and handed Jane the remote.

"Thanks," she said, the first word she had spoken since coming home.

She smiled halfheartedly and started clicking through the channels. Now that Jane was engrossed in TV, I tried to pause for a moment to get my bearings, but I couldn't—my thoughts raced in a thousand different directions. Rather than chasing after them, I distracted myself by tidying up the bedroom. As I folded Jane's clothes and put her shoes in the closet, I stole glances at her. Each time I did, all I could think was that, more than anything else in the world, I wanted our lives to go back to the way they were. Jane was home again so it was tempting to believe that it might be possible to turn back the clock. After all, she looked so normal lying in bed— the bedclothes did a great job of hiding the lumpy dressing over her tumor—I could almost fool myself into believing that this was just an ordinary Saturday afternoon with Jane watching television and me bustling around the apartment doing chores.

I couldn't sustain the illusion. The wheelchair in the corner of the bedroom, the noisy oxygen generator next to the bed, the tubing under Jane's nose—they were all too real to ignore. As much as I may have wanted to find it, there was no discernible path back to my old life. Until two weeks ago, I had been cosseted by comfortable routines evolved over thirty years of marriage and career. Now, with head-spinning rapidity, all that stability had been blown to bits.

What I was experiencing was hardly unique—plenty of families have had their lives upended by unforeseen medical catastrophes. But our cataclysm was *not* unforeseen—it had been deliberately hidden. I'm not suggesting that Jane's pulmonary embolus could have been predicted with certainty. Rather, had she shared her cancer diagnosis, we might, at the very least, have been prepared for the calamity. Even better, her doctors might have anticipated the possibility that she'd develop blood clots and tried to prevent them. Instead, because Jane chose secrecy and silence, she gave us no opportunity to plan together, to anticipate untoward events, to be ready for the illness we were now facing and the burden of her debility.

Those were my angry thoughts as I settled Jane into her bedroom. Their tinge of self-pity was intensified by my feeling that I was in this alone, that I had no one to talk with about what I was facing. But I realized that this negativity was not going to be particularly helpful, especially on my first night at home with Jane.

It also occurred to me that I wasn't as isolated as I thought. I still had our friends Michael and Christopher. Just thinking about them made me smile.

After Jane and Michael completed their fellowships and joined the faculty, Christopher, who had trained as an oncology fellow at a different hospital in Boston, joined his partner at Dana-Farber where they became the first guests at Jane's High Table. For nearly ten years, dinners with Michael and Christopher had been our sole social activity. This may have been a consequence, in part, of their being the only childless couple we knew and of Jane having rendered us functionally "childless" by her indifference to Anna. While the rest of our colleagues were busy having children or taking care of children or talking about taking care of children, the four of us gravitated toward each other.

But that wasn't what formed the basis of our friendship. Rather, from the moment we met, we knew that we had shared sensibilities. They were voracious readers, as were we, and our tastes were similar. Our opinions on career and colleagues, on politics and art, provided endless fodder for conversation. Michael was particularly close to Jane, who he referred to as his "surrogate sister."

In one area, however, we were only 75 percent aligned. Classical music had been a huge part of my life growing up and still is. Michael and Christopher were devotees, too, but they outdid me. I had always thought that my collection of classical LPs and CDs was impressive, but theirs dwarfed mine. Coincidentally, Christopher and I were both from Cleveland and worshipped the Cleveland Orchestra and the memory of George Szell, its legendary and terrifyingly autocratic conductor. We had both gone out of our way to acquire as much as we could from Szell's discography. Michael's appreciation was just as deep. I can still see him leaning back on the sofa, eyes half closed, conducting recordings with subtle movements of his hands.

Jane did not share this interest. In fact, she hated classical music. More particularly, she claimed that she couldn't stand the sound of the piano, which, of course, was my instrument. I told her once about a chamber music concert I'd heard in which the featured work was a piano quintet. Her eyes widened in horror.

"Five pianos? Are you kidding me? That's sheer torture!" she cried.

When I explained that piano quintets were made up of four string instruments—which she could tolerate—and only one piano, she was mollified, but just barely.

Who knows where her allergic reaction came from? Jane had taken violin lessons as a child but it had been an unhappy experience. She rarely practiced and would occasionally "forget" to bring her bow to a lesson. I think she told me once about a peeing episode during a recital. That might do it.

Undaunted by this misalignment, our friendship thrived. We spent countless hours together sharing the stories and confessions that distinguish intimates from acquaintances. By now, they knew Jane better than anyone who wasn't married to her. I needed to let them know what had happened.

My first impulse was to call Christopher—I thought he'd be better able to tell Michael about the horrible situation than I would—but I couldn't do it. Christopher was medically sophisticated. He'd want to know why Jane had had such a large pulmonary embolus. He'd know that advanced cancer is a common cause of blood clots and he'd certainly ask me about that. I knew that Jane wouldn't want me to reveal her secret. I also knew that I couldn't lie to Christopher. I was stuck.

Jane's demand that no one know about her history was one reason for not calling our friends, but another was that I didn't want to upset them. They so loved and admired Jane that, occasionally, they entertained an idealized image of her. Michael used to say that he pictured Jane as a tall, elegantly dressed woman, standing in front of an impressively stoked fireplace in an English drawing room, taking casual sips from her glass of Scotch whiskey. It hardly mattered that Jane hated standing, didn't like fires, and abhorred Scotch.

Despite the fact that "fantasy Jane" did not comport with "real Jane," I loved that Michael and Christopher saw her this way. I loved it enough that I did not want to tarnish Jane's image by revealing how we'd arrived at our current state. At least not yet—there'd be time for that later.

As I bustled around the bedroom, thinking of our friends, a call came from the lobby downstairs. It was the home health aide who had been sent to spend the night with us. I buzzed her in and told her to take the elevator to our floor. A few minutes later, Barbara knocked on the door. I was surprised by how happy I was to see her. Having someone else in the apartment—especially someone with actual expertise—felt like a gift.

At the same time, Barbara's presence put me on edge. Jane and I had spent decades living in our bubble. Between her desire to keep family at arm's length and our shared lack of interest in any sort of social life, we hardly ever invited people into our apartment other than Michael and Christopher. So, having a stranger there was as disconcerting as it was comforting.

My unease was worsened by my ignorance about how we were supposed to interact with her. Where exactly does she stay? Does she join us for dinner? How do I ask her to do things? *Do* I ask her to do things?

Fortunately, Barbara took charge. After making her introductions, she asked where the bedroom was. I showed her in. She introduced herself to Jane, had a quick conversation with her to make sure she didn't need anything, and then found her way back to the living room, where she commandeered an easy chair. Settling in, she rummaged around in a big canvas bag from which she retrieved two Tupperware bowls containing her dinner. Without much ado, she began to eat. Okay, then. I guess that's how we interact.

Seeing Barbara tuck in reminded me that it was suppertime. My usual Saturday routine was to go grocery shopping in the afternoon and use what I'd bought to make a nice dinner for Jane and me. That wouldn't be happening today. Our alternative—which we resorted to frequently—was to have food delivered from a restaurant. That seemed more practical under the circumstances.

I asked Jane which of our go-to neighborhood places she'd like me to order from. She said that she didn't care; the choice was mine. It didn't occur to me until later that I was being pretty insensitive—a bit of an idiot, really. Jane had just been released from the hospital where the dietitians had only slowly been advancing the amount of solid food she could tolerate in her meals.

It was no surprise, then, that she barely touched the deli food I ordered. This was an important lesson—I had to be more mindful that things were not normal and adjust my behavior accordingly. So, I made Jane some toast and served it with the only thing she ever drank at dinner anyway: a tall glass of Coke on ice. As a concession to her weakness, I added a bendy straw, something I'd had the foresight to include in my shopping spree from the day before. The dinner episode wasn't a major setback by any means—Jane was happy with the toast and Coke—but it was a harbinger of the way routines that we had established and come to rely upon were being altered or abandoned altogether.

Later in the evening, just before Jane was ready to go to sleep, Barbara got her out of bed and, with the help of a walker and some extra-long oxygen tubing, guided her to the bathroom. Later in the year, Jane would be reduced to using a bedside commode and ultimately a bedpan but, for now, she could take advantage of the raised toilet seat I had ordered for her. When she was finished, Barbara cleaned her and took her back to bed.

After Barbara returned to her station in the living room, I lay down on the bed next to Jane. We talked a little and watched TV together for an hour until she felt sleepy. I kissed her goodnight, then walked down the hall to the guest room and got into bed. I was comforted by the fact that Barbara was only twenty feet away and that the intercom connecting me to Jane's nightstand was within easy reach. Those reassuring thoughts lulled me to sleep on the first night of our new reality.

ELEVEN

When I awoke the next morning, my thoughts went right to the dauntingly elaborate surgical dressing covering Jane's tumor. It would have to be changed today. How exactly was I supposed to do that? I couldn't possibly manage it myself. Was anyone aware that I would need help?

Fortunately, the cavalry arrived promptly at eight o'clock. I'd been too sleep-deprived to remember that the home health care agency had, in fact, been informed that Jane's tumor would require daily nursing care and that they'd assigned us two visiting nurses who would alternate their coverage days. They showed up together on this first morning so we could meet them both.

Flo and Olivia had grown up in Revere, a working-class town just north of Boston known for its popular beach and its connection to organized crime. They were in the same class at Revere High (go Patriots!) and, after graduating, went to nursing school together. Now they worked for the agency providing our home care and, whenever possible, traded shifts with each other. That was a great strategy for them and provided continuity of care for their clients.

Flo was tough. She was built like a fireplug and wore heavy makeup featuring painted-on eyebrows. We learned later—from her—that her impressively ample bust had been surgically enhanced. Some Revere natives have a characteristic accent that makes anything they say sound vaguely threatening. Flo had that in spades—when she spoke, you listened.

I welcomed Flo's blustering authority. It was a relief to let her take charge of the nursing issues. She knew how to order all of the supplies we needed and would turn into a pitiless bloodhound if a shipment was late. Whenever her agency, which was headquartered in nearby Chelsea, failed to come through, she'd mutter, "Fuckin' Chelsea," nearly spitting out the second word so that it sounded like "TSCHELL-see!" Then she'd get on the phone and give her supervisors hell.

Flo took absolutely no guff from Eric or anyone else who formally outranked her in the medical hierarchy. She also made relentless fun of me.

"I gotta ask you," she'd say, "why do you leave your shoetrees on your bed in the other room?"

"I don't know," I answered. "I never really thought about it."

"I mean, who're you trying to impress? You want us all to know about your fancy Italian shoes? I can see 'em on your feet, you know... and my, my," she continued, pointing at my feet while casting a sidelong look at Jane, "aren't they fancy!"

Jane could barely suppress her laughter during these exchanges. An emotional alliance was being forged between Flo and Jane, one that made Jane feel like she had a fearless advocate.

Flo was clearly alpha dog but Olivia was hardly a pushover. She had a sweeter disposition but could be just as tough—she could spit out TSCHELL-see just like Flo when vexed by her bosses. And she was every bit as competent. Olivia also had no illusions about Flo—she would occasionally indulge in highly entertaining asides about her partner when she was with us on her own.

Both nurses were soon devoted to Jane. I watched her do the same thing with Flo and Olivia that she had done with countless trainees. She asked them about their lives, listened intently, and then gave them unambiguous advice, which was artfully embedded in funny and entertaining commentary. Jane learned all she could about their families and their romances. There seemed to be an unending stream of idiot brothers, sketchy but loving boyfriends, overbearing mothers, and beloved grandmothers. Jane remembered everyone's name and where they fit in the Revere tapestry. This wasn't just some parlor trick—she was genuinely interested. The result was two more people who would walk through fire for Jane.

Of course, our light-hearted banter was framed by the grim reality of Jane's tumor. That was the anchor around which all other activities were organized. The mass secreted copious amounts of a serum-like fluid which, after a while, would make the dressings so uncomfortably wet that they'd have to be changed once or, eventually, twice a day. All other concerns were secondary.

We had a rhythm. At eight o'clock on the dot, one of the nurses—let's say Flo—presses the button on our building's intercom to let us know that she's in the lobby. I buzz her in, and while she rides the elevator to our floor, I grab a trash bag from the kitchen and take it into Jane's bedroom, opening the apartment door for Flo along the way and leaving it ajar. If Jane's not awake yet, I gently nudge her and whisper that Flo's here. As I loop the edge of the garbage bag over the post at the foot of the bed, I hear Flo's clogs coming down the hall.

Flo bounds into the bedroom, says good morning to Jane, and gives her a hug. She checks Jane's vital signs and tells her about the latest troubles with her fiancé. Meanwhile, I spread an absorbent pad on the bed at Jane's feet—this will be my work area—and assemble the things we'll need for the dressing change:

- A wide Ace bandage
- A narrow Ace bandage
- Two sets of sterile surgical gloves
- Three large gauze dressings infused with petroleum jelly (these are usually used for burns—the brand name is Xeroform)
- Four large absorbent gauze pads (known as ABD pads)

- Two rolls of crinkly gauze (brand name Kerlix)
- Several four-inch-by-four-inch gauze pads
- Three large Stayfree Maxi pads—the yellow ones—opened and sitting on their wrappers
- Rolls of paper tape
- Sharp scissors
- A tube of triple antibiotic ointment
- Coagulation strips or silver nitrate–tipped wooden sticks to stop any bleeding we might encounter

When Jane's ready, Flo and I sit her up and untie her johnnie, lowering it to her waist. The only thing visible below Jane's bare shoulders is a large Ace bandage that's wrapped twice around her torso and a narrow Ace bandage that runs over her right shoulder. It occurs to me that this is what Jane would look like if she were binding her chest.

I remove the narrow bandage over Jane's right shoulder. If it's dry, we'll use it again; if it's wet, it goes in the laundry. Then I start unrolling the large bandage around her chest, checking carefully to see if it's been stained by liquid or blood that may have seeped through the deeper layers of the dressing during the night. Jane desperately hates to see or feel any dampness on her dressing. Whenever she's awake, she repeatedly asks, "Am I wet?" and orders me to check the bandage. So, even the slightest discoloration or dampness relegates it to the laundry basket.

With the Ace bandages removed, I can see the next layer of the dressing: two rolls of crinkly Kerlix gauze wrapped around Jane's chest. The Kerlix keeps the rest of the bulky dressing in place, so removing it requires careful choreography. I stabilize the dressing with one hand and use the other to gather up both rolls of Kerlix and toss them into the trash. Then, with one hand still on the dressing, Flo and I gently lower Jane onto her back. As we do so, we slide absorbent pads underneath her to soak up any liquid that may run down her side later.

Maxi pads make up the next layer. They were a brilliant suggestion from Sue the surgeon to address Jane's phobia about wet dressings. These things were specifically designed to absorb liquid and keep women dry, she said, so why not use them here? They were amazingly effective. I lift them up and, as I do, their adhesive undersurface brings up the ABD pads that form the layer below. The whole mess is sopping wet from the tumor and goes into the trash. Now the Xeroform—the petroleum jelly–containing gauze—is exposed. It's the final layer, the one directly on top of the tumor. I take my time peeling back the Xeroform, making sure that it isn't stuck to any of the dead tissue on the tumor's surface. If I'm not fastidious about this, the Xeroform can lift away some of the tumor's superficial layers and cause bleeding. Finally, if I had placed gauze "flowers"—another learning from Sue—into the crevasses of Jane's tumor during the previous dressing change, I remove them with care.

Now Jane's chest is fully exposed. Flo and I can see if there are any bleeding sites in the main mass and whether any new satellite tumors may have appeared. Most important, we can see if there's any redness extending from the tumor onto Jane's normal skin. This is our best indicator of infection.

Flo cleans the tumor mass using a spray of sterile saline and then gently pats it dry with gauze. If there are nooks or crannies in the tumor that would benefit from stanching, I make some fresh gauze flowers and insert them into those troublesome areas, using the tip of a forceps. Flo then picks up a new Xeroform dressing by its edges and I squeeze a healthy amount of antibiotic ointment over its surface. She folds the Xeroform on itself to spread the antibiotic, then opens it up again and lays it across the upper half of the tumor, pressing here and there to make sure it conforms to the shape of the mass. Then we do the same thing over the lower half so that the entire tumor is covered with Xeroform. Sometimes, when the nurses can't come to the apartment, I have to do the Xeroform prep myself, which is impossibly awkward. Things always go better when I have a partner, mostly for the dressing mechanics but also for engaging in some back and forth—reliably starting with Flo making fun of me—that distracts Jane. Later in the year, when we were doing twice-daily dressing changes, I had no choice. I was always alone for the evening change and would have to handle the Xeroform and antibiotic myself.

By now my gloves are covered with petroleum jelly and antibiotic ointment, making it impossible to grip anything, so I take them off, toss them into the trash, and put on a fresh pair. Using my new gloves, I place one ABD pad over the Xeroform at the top of Jane's tumor and secure it to her chest with paper tape. I place two more ABD pads over the rest of the Xeroform, making my way down the tumor by overlapping the edges of the ABDs like shingles. Next come the maxi pads. I place three large ones in an overlapping pattern over the ABD pads.

The only way to keep this ungainly mass of cotton, paper, and plastic in place is to wrap Jane's chest. This also requires careful maneuvering. Flo and I gently sit Jane up while holding the dressing material in place. Then I slide one end of a Kerlix roll under the hand stabilizing the dressing and unroll it against Jane's chest. There's enough material in one roll to make it around her chest twice, which allows me to tuck the free end under the Kerlix itself to hold it in place. It's not enough coverage, so I have to wrap her with a second Kerlix roll, but this is easier to do since the first one is partially retaining the dressing.

Jane had some small satellite tumor masses near her right shoulder that also had to be covered with Xeroform and gauze. Because they were outside of the main dressing, we devised a different system to hold these materials in place. Our solution involved draping a narrow Ace bandage over Jane's right shoulder, like a bandolier. That secured things.

With the dressing's main components finally in place, the last step is to lock it all down by winding a large Ace bandage twice around Jane's chest. This is yet another delicate procedure since the Ace has to be snug enough to keep the dressing in place but not so tight that it restricts Jane's breathing. It was not uncommon to have to rewrap the Ace two or three times before Jane was comfortable.

At that point I remove the full and foul-smelling garbage bag from the bedpost and put it in the trash. We joke a little with Flo and then she leaves.

The next morning we do it again.

Although we rarely encountered any surprises—every step had been routinized—and we tried to keep the mood light, the dressing changes were traumatic for Jane. The secret she had hidden for so long was now exposed every day while she lay helpless in bed.

The dressing changes were traumatic for me too. The setting created a grotesque intimacy in which I gazed at and touched Jane's bare chest, including her normal left breast. I had been forced into the role of a medical provider, but I was also Jane's husband, and we had shared intimate memories and feelings about her nakedness that had nothing at all to do with illness. I didn't know what to do with those thoughts. Mostly I walled them off.

Often, when we had removed the previous day's dressing and Jane's tumor was fully exposed, I found myself alternating between seeing it as part of Jane, which was horrifying, and as something totally separate, its own object. My reification of the cancer was clearly self-protective, but it ran the risk of objectifying Jane too.

As time went on, though, the idea of Jane's tumor being an integral part of her began to lose its power to horrify. Somehow—through compassion, I suppose—I found a way of feeling terribly sad about her cancer and impending death without experiencing the knee-jerk revulsion that the tumor itself had first caused. And despite all of my worries about falling into the trap of turning Jane into a mere object, of no longer connecting to her emotionally, it never happened.

TWELVE

Each dressing change consumed an impressive amount of sterile paper, plastic, cotton, and maxi pads. Having everything we needed every day of every week of every month created logistic challenges, but Flo and Olivia were on it, anticipating when we were about to run out of supplies and ordering more from the agency. As a result, we'd get huge boxes delivered to our apartment two or three times a week. We had a large Jacuzzi in our bathroom—installed by the previous owner, not really our thing—and we used it to store all of the stuff we needed for Jane's dressing changes. It was filled to the brim. Our bathroom looked like the stockroom of a medical supply store.

The only thing the agency did not supply was maxi pads. The first few times I went to the drugstore to buy six boxes of large feminine hygiene pads, I was embarrassed. I kept wondering what the checkout person was thinking. After a while, my maxi pad runs became routine and I didn't give them a second thought. Eventually, though, I wised up and ordered them in bulk from Amazon. My maxi pad preferences are now embedded in one of their algorithms.

Another glancing blow to my masculinity occurred about halfway through the year when Jane started entertaining thoughts of going back to work. Her main concern wasn't whether she'd have enough physical strength; she was worried about her appearance. In particular, she thought that the bulky dressing over her right-sided tumor mass would make her chest look lopsided. Jane was not particularly

94

large-breasted, and she thought she needed some kind of enhancement on the left to balance things.

So, Jane patiently taught me about silicone wedges—known as
"cutlets," she said—that could do the trick by fitting into a bra cup. My
job was to try to find them. Several department stores were within
walking distance of our Back Bay apartment. Again, I squelched
my embarrassment and visited the women's lingerie department at
each one.

The nice lady at Neiman Marcus looked like she was going to call
security as she pointedly told me that they didn't have what I was
looking for. The salesperson at Lord & Taylor was more sympathetic
but also couldn't help. I struck gold at Saks and cleaned out their
supply of four cutlets. I silently apologized to all the other women of
Boston who might have been looking for a non-surgical boost.

It was Christmas time, so, as long as I was there, I thought I
would get Jane a present. I decided on a new robe that she could
wear over her sad hospital gown. When the salesperson asked what
size I needed, I said I wasn't sure. But Jane and I were almost exactly
the same height, so I took off my suit jacket—I had come from work—
and slipped on the robe. There I was, standing in Saks Fifth Avenue
wearing a lovely lady's bathrobe while holding four breast-enhanc-
ing cutlets in my hand. Not for the first or last time, I muttered to
myself, "How exactly did this happen?"

In fact, my commitment to caring for Jane in all things was
nothing new. I had devoted the past thirty years to her, after all, but
it hadn't been easy. To sustain a marriage for that long, couples must
decide to accept or at least tolerate their partners' annoying tics.
Healthy couples talk about these little aggravations and together
figure out ways to live with them. Other couples avoid confrontation
and try instead to suppress their annoyance in the belief that not
having difficult conversations is the same thing as happiness. We
were all-in for the latter.

Between the decision not to have children of our own and my capitulation to Jane's wish to keep Anna at a distance, we had established an early pattern of exclusive reliance on each other. Ours was a fundamentally emotional interdependence, but it had very practical results. Because Jane was convinced that she could not drive a car—she thought she was too poorly coordinated and too easily distractible—I took her everywhere. This wasn't much of a burden. I liked the fact that we drove together to work every morning and home every night.

But being an on-call chauffeur was nothing compared with the more serious challenges that arose from Jane's addictive tendencies. Her smoking habit, later supplanted by her Nicorette habit, was an obvious manifestation, but there were others.

For the first few years we were together, she kept packs of playing cards in strategic locations throughout the apartment—all within easy reach for endless games of solitaire. Whenever she was in bed, for example, she would turn on the television, grab a deck, and start playing. It took real persuading to get her to put down the cards and go to sleep. Whenever she was at her desk, she would turn on a small portable television and start dealing herself solitaire hands. A few years later, Jane bought a personal computer so that she could play computer games instead of solitaire. Tetris—two-dimensional, then three-dimensional—Minesweeper, FreeCell (of course), it didn't matter. There must have been other people who devoted hours to those games, but I know of no one else who could wake up on Saturday morning, plop herself in front of a vintage PC, start playing Tetris, not stop until bedtime, then wake up on Sunday and do it again.

I watched helplessly as this behavior gradually intensified. Eventually, she would stay up until four in the morning on weekends playing computer games; sometimes she wouldn't go to bed at all. On weekdays, she would make a beeline for her computer as soon as we got home. I would have to raise my voice to get her to stop long enough to have dinner with me. As soon as she was done eating, she was back at the PC. I finally gave up and figured that Jane would join me when she joined me, whether it was at the dinner table or in bed.

I briefly entertained the notion that Jane was using her behavior to avoid spending time with me, but for reasons of self-preservation, I convinced myself that wasn't the case. I even had some evidence to support this inference. When we were on vacation, for example, and Jane didn't have access to her computer, she happily stayed right by my side. Perhaps I was deluded but I always thought that, fundamentally, she loved me and loved my company, and that this was all about something else, not me.

In fact, I have neither the insight nor the clinical expertise to understand the meaning of Jane's compulsive and solitary game-playing. Some of her family members, recalling how she behaved as a child and observing her fidgeting as an adult, have wondered if she might have been on the high-functioning end of the autism spectrum. I don't think that's the case. She was far too adept at interpreting the most subtle of social cues for this to be a tenable diagnosis.

Whatever the precise nature of her underlying psychology might have been, my guess is that Jane used these behaviors to tamp down anxiety. I wasn't always aware of the source of her fears—her illness phobia only became fully apparent later—but I sympathized with their impact. I knew how my own anxiety disorder could make me feel, so I tended to give Jane all the space she needed for her fidgety countermeasures no matter how annoying or alienating I found them.

* * *

The practical outcome of Jane's refusal to drive, her tendency to procrastinate, and her proclivity for being immobile when she was home—except for fingers moving on a keyboard—was that the household chores fell to me. All of them. I did the laundry and the grocery shopping, I managed our finances, I prepared our meals, I took out the garbage. Jane was supposed to wash the dinner dishes but needed regular reminders and cajoling. Even then, she only did it half the time.

I have no doubt that Jane appreciated all of the many things I did for her. I had heard from her coworkers that Jane would admit, somewhat sheepishly, that she knew she had been lucky to find someone who was willing to make her life so easy. Other times, she'd brag about how she had found the "perfect husband" and then list all of the chores I took responsibility for. For some reason she associated this trait with being Jewish and would tell her friends that the best thing they could ever do for themselves would be to "marry a Jewish man."

Her comments made me uncomfortable. I couldn't be sure that Jane might not have harbored a little disrespect for my readiness to take on the household tasks—that, while appreciating how obliging I was, she might also think I was being weak for rolling over so easily. And it's not as if I didn't have my own ambivalence about catering to Jane's needs. On one hand, I derived tremendous satisfaction from taking care of her, and she was usually good about showing her appreciation. On the other, either because she hadn't acknowledged something I'd done for her or because I was just feeling put upon, my frustration could boil over.

I remember a Saturday afternoon early in our relationship when, after I had done the grocery shopping and served Jane both her breakfast and lunch in bed, I was ready to take care of some personal priority. Jane chose that precise moment to ask me to do yet one more thing that she reasonably could have done herself. Instead of asking her to do it instead, I grumbled my assent. As I walked out of the bedroom, I angrily kicked the wall. I had done this a few times before but, on this occasion, my foot went right through the drywall. I was thoroughly embarrassed that I had let my anger get the best of me. And, of course, I paid for it by spending my Saturday afternoon spackling.

I think my reaction scared Jane a little. For years afterward, when she thought she might be demanding a little too much, she would ask, "You're not going to kick the wall, are you?" There were probably less destructive ways to put limits on her requests but this one worked for a while.

Now that Jane was mortally ill, though, accommodating her needs took on a different meaning. There was no room for resentment. Sadness and pity colored my response to new "demands" like insisting that I stand by in case she needed help while trying to take a shower or washing her hair on her own instead of being bathed by Barbara. Having some autonomy, even in this narrow domain, probably gave Jane the sense that she was still in control of her life. I had been dimly aware of this need and had tried to anticipate it. One of the items I had snagged at Bed Bath & Beyond was a hand-held shower head, which I had installed in the master bath. I'd also ordered a plastic seat from a medical supply company so that Jane wouldn't have to stand while using it.

What I hadn't foreseen was that we would have to find a way to keep the bulky dressing over Jane's tumor from getting wet. Barbara came up with a brilliant idea. She cut a head-sized hole in the bottom of a plastic kitchen garbage bag and then had Jane sit on the chair in the shower while she lowered the bag over her head, guiding it through the hole. Barbara then pulled the rest of the bag down to cover Jane's shoulders and chest. Now Jane could shampoo her hair without soaking the dressing.

Ordinarily, Barbara would help Jane but, on demand, the task would fall to me. My job was to help Jane get in and out of the shower and to stay in the bathroom with her while she washed herself in case she needed anything.

After guiding Jane to the seat in in the shower stall and turning on the water, I would close the door and lean against the opposite wall, waiting for her to finish. Our shower door was glass, so I would spend ten minutes or so with nowhere to look but at my wife, naked save for her trash bag. After ten years of living with an inadequately treated breast cancer, her physical wasting had become profound. She seemed to have no muscle mass at all—she was all sagging skin and sharply protruding bones. She looked so exposed and so weak. It was a reminder of where this was all heading.

THIRTEEN

Once the dressing changes became routine, I thought things might be stable enough for me to go back to work. After all, Barbara would be home with Jane in case anything happened. So, I created a new schedule for myself. After the dressing change was done and the nurses had left, I'd check to make sure Jane had whatever she needed by her bedside. Then I'd kiss her, tell her I loved her, and head for the Farber. I was surprised by how easy it was to put what was happening at home in its own compartment so that I could be productive at the hospital.

One morning, though, about six weeks after Jane had come home, something did happen. Jane called me at work.

"I'm bleeding," she said.

I thought back to the episode on the bathroom floor four years earlier when she'd spoken the same words in the same emotionless way.

"From where?" I asked, opting for the persona of objective physician rather than worried spouse.

"From the tumor. Where else?" she said. "It's not stopping."

"Okay," I said, now feeling worried. "I can be home in ten minutes."

"No, this is bad," she said with a new hint of panic in her voice. "I've already called 911. An ambulance is coming to take me to the emergency room at the Brigham."

"Okay, good," I said. "I'll meet you there. How are you doing?"

"I'm worried."

"Me too, but you're doing the right thing. You'll be in good hands as soon as the EMTs arrive and I'll see you at the Brigham."

"Wait. It sounds like they're here."

I could hear the siren over the phone. The bedroom windows must have been open.

"Perfect. See you right away."

She hung up.

Jane had a very specific fear about bleeding from her tumor. It was the bleeding, more than anything else, that had compelled her to reveal her secret to me on the bathroom floor. Her fear had only intensified since then. Now, every time we exposed the tumor during a dressing change, she would anxiously ask, "Do you see blood?" In between dressing changes, if she felt any moisture at all on the Ace bandage around her chest, she would look at me with terror in her eyes and say, "What's that? Is it blood?"

Her concern was rational. The pulmonary embolus that had nearly killed her was caused by a blood clot that traveled to her lungs from the veins in her legs. The reason it had formed in the first place was because of her underlying disease. As long as Jane still had her breast cancer, she would be at risk of developing another clot. Something had to be done to try to keep that from happening.

The standard approach to preventing blood clots is to administer medications that inhibit the clotting process, drugs known colloquially as blood thinners. However, Jane's enormous tumor was fed by an irregular system of fragile blood vessels that were prone to leakage, which could cause spontaneous bleeding. The tumor had also eroded into some of the normal blood vessels in the skin and muscles of her chest—that was the cause of the episode on the bathroom floor. The only thing keeping Jane from bleeding to death from either source was her blood's ability to clot. So, Eric, as her oncologist, had to strike a balance between suppressing Jane's clotting strongly enough to prevent another pulmonary embolus but not so strongly that she would bleed uncontrollably from her tumor.

Anti-clotting drugs come in different varieties, each with its own properties. Eric decided to give Jane a short-acting formulation of a standard medication called heparin so that its effects would wear off quickly if her tumor were to bleed. The problem was that it couldn't be taken orally—it had to be injected. I had intended to foist this responsibility onto Flo and Olivia since I was already making myself—and Jane—uncomfortable by playing such a prominent role in the dressing changes. I thought that adding heparin shots to my list of daily tasks would only further muddy the distinction between husband and caregiver.

But Jane needed her heparin every day—it was lifesaving—and she would need it even if Flo or Olivia weren't available. So, the heparin injections became my job after all. I just steeled myself and tried to be gentle when I jabbed sharp needles into the skin of my wife's abdomen every morning. The other consequence of daily heparin shots was that the medical stockroom in our Jacuzzi now held boxes of pre-loaded heparin syringes, alcohol swabs, and bio-hazard containers for the disposal of used needles.

I'll confess that, despite my medical training, being in charge of the heparin injections made me uncomfortable. I was constantly worried that I was hurting Jane—that I was making my own per-sonal contribution to her misery. At first, I did see her wince every time I poked her. Thankfully, my technique improved. One of the sweetest things Jane ever said to me was that I was better at giving her heparin shots than anyone else. I'm an incurable romantic.

For the most part, the short-acting heparin did its job. Occasion-ally, however, the delicate balance it was supposed to strike between clotting and bleeding could tip in the wrong direction. That's what had happened today.

I dropped what I was doing and walked quickly to the ER—by now I knew the way. I got there just as the EMTs were rolling Jane's stretcher into one of the examination rooms. Jane's fear of a major hemorrhage had worked her into a full-blown panic attack, but a quick assessment by one of the residents revealed that the bleeding was actually minor.

When the resident was finished, the director of the ER came into the room to evaluate Jane. He gently probed the tumor and pointed to one or two spots where small amounts of blood were still oozing. He had been an army physician and told Jane that, in the field, he used to treat bleeding wounds with strips of cloth that were impregnated with something that causes instantaneous clotting. He asked a nurse to retrieve a packet of these magic strips. She disappeared for a minute and then returned carrying a small box, which she handed to the doctor. He used a forceps to pull a strip from the box and cut it into small pieces, which he wedged into the areas of the tumor he was concerned about. Poof—the bleeding stopped.

Jane was beside herself with excitement—the strips had not only stopped the bleeding, they had dispelled her panic. The ER doctor smiled at Jane's reaction and gave us the rest of the packet to take home. I called Flo right away and asked her to put a box of these clotting strips in our next supply order. She called me back a few hours later to say that the agency wouldn't provide them—"fuckin' TSCHELL-see." Apparently, they were too exotic to be covered by our insurance.

It was a long shot, but I checked Amazon. Perhaps I shouldn't have been surprised to see that I could order battlefield trauma supplies at reasonable prices. Two boxes arrived a few days later. Now, whenever we saw bleeding from Jane's tumor during a dressing change, I could apply the strips, just like the ER doctor did, and make it stop. This was a triumph. I only used them rarely, but just knowing that they were an arm's length away on Jane's dresser was enough to assuage her fears.

* * *

It was one thing to treat Jane's bleeding, quite another to treat her underlying cancer. Any approach Eric might take would be confounded by Jane's years-long history of hiding her disease and treating it herself. His planning would be further affected by her complicated thoughts about being a cancer patient.

Initially, I had assumed that Jane's sole rationale for her secrecy was denial. Acknowledging her cancer would have made it—and the suffering and death it would inevitably cause—far too real. Better to tell no one and not have to think about it.

But that's an overly facile explanation for the behavior of someone as sophisticated as Jane. Instead—or, perhaps, in addition—it was vitally important to her not to be seen as a cancer patient. This may seem like an odd worry, especially for an oncologist, but there were at least two reasons for her concern.

First, Jane had seen the way attitudes abruptly shift when people learn that someone has cancer—the newly diagnosed suddenly find themselves approached by others with a condescending mixture of indulgence and pity. Jane prided herself on her toughness, and she had always been deeply insecure about being perceived as weak. Those fears still tortured her—she could not tolerate the aura of frailty and vulnerability that would have accompanied her public transformation into "a person with cancer."

Second, Jane did not want to be associated with a stereotype that's used so often to describe cancer patients, especially those with breast cancer: The Brave Fighter. The label was anathema to her. Jane had been contemptuously critical of the attitude of advocates, support groups, family members, and oncologists who, in her opinion, shamed patients into declaring, "I'm going to fight this thing!" Jane understood that the disease was implacable—metastatic breast cancer cannot be cured. She thought that fooling patients into thinking they had agency when they had none was irresponsible. It could only lead to feelings of failure when, through no fault of their own, their breast cancers became resistant to all therapies and eventually killed them. Jane wanted no part of that.

I have sympathy for her stance, one that's consistent with the piti-lessly objective side of her personality. In fact, I'm pretty sure that I would have been a willing co-conspirator if Jane had explained her decision to me this way. I would have kept her secret and, perhaps, been better prepared to care for her during her final months. But she didn't give me the chance.

Is it fair for me to blame Jane for her own misery? Can I say that by not fully confiding in me, Jane prevented me from helping her? Maybe. But maybe the truth is that I didn't push hard enough and, in that way, I failed her. Something had been wrong with her for nearly ten years and, for four of those years, I knew that it was breast cancer—at least that's what she said it was. I did make a few half-hearted attempts to convince her to seek medical attention, but each one ended in tears and a demand that I never mention it again. So, I backed off.

Even if I had continued to press her, there's no guarantee that I could ever have convinced Jane to see a doctor. But what if I had? Would she have lived longer? Probably not. Her breast cancer was so far advanced, even when she first told me about it, that treatment was not likely to give her more years of life.

But the value that an individual places on her life is not deter-mined solely by its length. Jane's own research had shown that other components of a life can be just as important as years of survival—sometimes more so. And their relative importance can vary from person to person. Jane often pointed out that when you consider the negative values that some people assign to certain types of debility—paralysis, dementia, chronic pain—you discover that merely dying is not the worst outcome they can imagine. She liked to remind oncol-ogists that there are states of health worse than death.

So, ironically, Jane's decision-making about her own cancer dovetailed with her research. One of her most important findings was that oncologists can be guilty of prescribing highly toxic but ineffective chemotherapy for patients with incurable cancers even if those patients may not want it. She had identified this problem by asking patients themselves what they understood about the therapy they were receiving and what their actual preferences were. She found that most weren't aware that their treatments were likely to be futile.

Jane's engagement with this research question had an emotional origin. She had seen firsthand the suffering that chemotherapy inflicted on dying cancer patients, largely to no avail. It horrified her. The toxicities were bad enough but, by focusing so intently on cancer treatment, doctors were keeping patients from having honest and useful discussions about their end-of-life preferences. Jane wouldn't want that for herself and she was pretty sure that, if patients were asked, they would say that they wouldn't want it either. Her data showed that she was right.

Ironically, Jane's research paper documenting how most patients with advanced cancer don't understand that the chemotherapy they're getting won't cure them was published in *The New England Journal of Medicine* the month after she had her pulmonary embolus, just as she was considering therapy for her own advanced cancer. Her work caught the attention of the popular press, and a reporter from the *New York Times* interviewed Jane on her sickbed. The article quoted her:

> *It's completely understandable that patients want to believe the chemo will cure them. And it's understandable that physicians hesitate to take away that false hope.... [But, if] patients think chemo has a chance of curing them, they'll be less likely to have end-of-life discussions early on and they pay a price for that later.*

It came as no surprise, then, that Jane refused standard chemotherapy. Eric tried only once to convince her that he could prevent, or at least mitigate, the toxicities. But Jane made her preferences clear, and he never brought it up again.

* * *

Despite Jane's reluctance to be perceived as a cancer patient, that is, of course, what she was. And, like all cancer patients, everything she experienced during her last year—the transient joys and the more lasting disappointments—took place against the backdrop of her cancer treatment. It was the ever-present theme that commanded our attention no matter what else was going on. Our lives were ruled by its unforgiving cycles—choosing a therapy, cautious optimism as it seemed to work, disenchantment when it inevitably failed, then the struggle to pick another from a narrowing list of options.

At first, I wasn't sure that Jane would let Eric treat her at all. Between her personal aversion to medical care and her general critique of useless cancer therapies, I thought she might refuse any treatment. But given her history of prescribing mild chemotherapy for herself, it seemed possible that she'd be willing to tolerate some sort of intervention as long as it came with minimal side effects. She was aware that nothing would cure her but, without treatment, the cancer was making her feel awful—she was fatigued, short of breath, and experiencing relentless pain in her chest and bones. Perhaps something tolerable might shrink her tumors enough to make her feel better, at least temporarily.

Eric's initial suggestion was for Jane to continue the oral chemotherapy she had started on her own. He thought it might provide palliation without causing serious side effects, and this time it would be safe because he'd be monitoring her blood counts. Jane accepted.

Once Jane was officially on therapy, I looked for ways to gauge its efficacy. I started by monitoring the size of the small tumors in her skin adjacent to the main mass. At every dressing change, I tried to determine if they had grown, shrunk, or stayed the same. But I had to be surreptitious. Rather than standing over Jane with a tape measure, I just kind of eyeballed them. I didn't want to draw attention to what I was doing because I didn't want to seem too invested in the success of her treatment knowing that, ultimately, it would fail.

Every so often, though, Jane would catch me looking at the tumors and ask, "What do you think? Are they getting bigger or smaller?" and I would answer honestly. When they were smaller, Jane would nod and say, "Good."

Later, when I had to tell her that they had grown bigger, she remained silent.

FOURTEEN

As fall turned to early winter, Jane began eating more and could even get out of bed for a while, if only to sit at her desk to play computer games. Along with her physical improvement, Jane's head had cleared—no more of that intense déjà vu she experienced after leaving the ICU—and, although she occasionally had bad dreams or intrusive thoughts about her time in intensive care, she mostly seemed to be her old self.

By November, Jane was looking so much better that I thought she might be able to enjoy one of our longstanding traditions: Thanksgiving dinner for two. Our chronic antisocial attitude usually forestalled invitations to join others for the holiday and we almost never had anyone to our place. Instead, I would spend the day cooking a complete Thanksgiving dinner just for Jane and me. She loved it, and I thoroughly enjoyed my time in the kitchen. So, I asked her if she'd like to give it a try. She said she would.

Although I'd always known how to cook a little, it had only recently become a real interest. That was all thanks to Christopher, who was my first foodie. I'm still in awe of the dinner he made for us when Michael and Jane were fellows. In those early days, our friends lived in a railroad apartment, within earshot of the expressway, in one of Boston's sketchier neighborhoods. The place was small—the dining room table spilled into the hallway—and the minuscule kitchen had only rudimentary appliances. Somehow, Christopher transcended these obstacles to prepare one of the best meals I'd ever had before

or since: a savory soup, a perfect main course with ideally comple-
mentary sides, and a fancy dessert, all accompanied by impressive
wines. I had no idea that a mere civilian could do something like
that. It was eye-opening.

Christopher's dinner took on new relevance a few years later
when I was cycling through one of my periods of professional
despondency—my work was pointless, I would never succeed, I was
a talentless hack, and so on. One day, near my nadir, I showed up late
for lunch. Apparently, my wife and friends had been sitting together
for a while. As I took my place, I glanced up to see that all three were
looking at me with conspiratorial grins.

"Barrett," Michael started. "We know what your problem is, and
we have a solution."

"Yes," Christopher continued. "You need a hobby. We've been
discussing it and we think that cooking would be the ideal distraction for you."

Jane remained silent but was clearly enjoying herself.

I was furious. Actually, first, I was embarrassed to be called out
for my pouty behavior. But then I was furious that my so-called
friends were trying to manage my life.

"Fuck you all," I said loudly enough to turn heads at nearby tables.
"Don't you dare patronize me."

"My good man!" said Michael, patting my hand. "We were only
trying to help!"

The rest of the meal passed in silence while I wallowed in my
sour mood.

The upshot, of course, was that I quietly began buying Julia Child
cookbooks, subscribing to *Bon Appétit*, and hanging out at Wil-
liams-Sonoma drooling over beautiful cookware. I learned to make
a few things and was surprised by how much I enjoyed the process.
Eventually, the co-conspirators forced me to admit that they'd been
right. Of course, by signing on to Christopher and Michael's suggestion, Jane had made herself the main beneficiary of my new hobby;

she became the recipient of an endless string of good meals willingly made, including holiday feasts.

Preparing things that Jane liked to eat was one of the ways I could show my affection for her. She once tried to return the compliment. For my sixtieth birthday—just a few months before her collapse— she sneaked into the kitchen after I had gone to bed the night before and baked a cake in the shape of a heart. She wrote, "I adore you," in red icing on the top.

This was a wonderful surprise but also a huge shock. Jane had never used our oven and confessed later that she didn't even know how to turn it on. After fiddling with the controls in the middle of the night for what seemed like an eternity, she thought she had it figured out and put the cake in the oven. When she took it out forty-five minutes later, it hadn't baked at all and the oven was suspiciously cold. Instead of pressing the "On" button, she had set the timer to turn on the oven twelve hours later. So, she threw out the old cake, mixed a new one, set the oven correctly, and baked a second cake at 4:00 a.m.

This was an astounding effort for someone who didn't cook and rarely even got out of bed. Also, by this time, Jane was becoming weaker and suffering from shortness of breath with the slightest exertion. When I shuffled bleary-eyed into the kitchen on my birth-day morning, I was flabbergasted to find the cake sitting on the breakfast table. The fact that it tasted horrendously bad—not knowing where I kept the cooking supplies, she had found a bottle of rancid oil—made no difference. The picture I took of the cake and its message is one of my prized possessions.

* * *

I got up early on Thanksgiving day raring to go. Of course, this year things would be different. Instead of heading straight for the kitchen, I started the day by giving Jane her heparin injection and helping Flo's holiday substitute with the dressing change. But after that, I was back in the saddle. By late afternoon, I had prepared a small turkey along with stuffing, mashed potatoes, green beans, and a pie. I was looking forward to a great holiday dinner followed by four days of leftovers.

I called to Jane, letting her know that the food was ready and that I would be in to help her walk to the dining room in a minute. I hadn't checked on her since the morning's medical activities so I was taken aback when, as I was laying out the food, I looked up and saw Jane, leaning on her walker, coming to the table under her own steam. She was wearing jeans, a blouse, and a red sweater. This was the first time I had seen her dressed in normal clothes since the day of her collapse. I gave her a hug, helped her sit down, and then ran back to the kitchen, where I stifled my sobs in a dish towel. It was overwhelming to see her looking so normal. It reminded me of just how much we had lost and still had to lose.

I collected myself and came back to the table. I served small portions of everything to Jane, and we began our dinner. But, after a few minutes, she said she couldn't eat any more and needed to go back to bed. She was panting a little and looked exhausted. I hadn't realized how much effort she'd expended just to try to have a normal evening. That was her gift to me.

From then on, Jane's difficulty with food grew worse. I'd try to entice her to eat more by making her favorite meals and she would gamely try, but her attempts generally ended in disaster. Sometimes she would vomit everything up an hour later. Other times, I'd get a panicked call on the intercom in the middle of the night to take her to the bathroom because of diarrhea. On at least one occasion, she called me too late and I had to clean her up and strip the bed. I'm surely not the first and won't be the last husband who tends to a sick wife who shits herself. I can only assume we've all felt the same confusing mix of revulsion, pity, and tenderness.

I finally gave up. By March, about six months after coming home from the hospital, the only food Jane could tolerate was Stouffer's frozen macaroni and cheese. I made it for her twice a day, every day, and served it up with her usual glass of Coke. She could usually eat only half. Thank goodness she could tolerate at least that much and never grew tired of it. But good god, I would think, look what she's been reduced to.

FIFTEEN

From the moment Jane regained consciousness in the ICU, she fought as hard as she could not to appear vulnerable. Her fear of being weak—or being perceived as such—was deeply ingrained. It had informed her behavior at the start of our relationship and it was still driving her now that she was objectively, incontrovertibly helpless. When I told her that I had asked Eric to be her oncologist, she was furious.

"How could you do that?" she asked with a look of incredulity. "What were you thinking?"

"Excuse me, but I was thinking that he's the best breast cancer doctor in Boston," I said. "What's the problem?"

"Yes, okay, fine," she said, shaking her head, "but I would never have wanted him to see me like this. Better to have someone who didn't know me."

"Even at the cost of that 'someone' not being as experienced or skilled in complicated cases like yours?"

"Yes. I don't see what the big deal is."

Well, that was a huge slug of denial, I thought, mixed with disgust at finding herself in a weak, dependent position.

Although I sympathized with Jane's struggles about her new reality, I also knew that she'd have to relent. At some point—soon, I hoped—she'd have to come to terms with the fact that she was a cancer patient whose treatment would now be directed by someone other than herself. She'd have to relinquish control.

Jane was, I knew, capable of softening. As I thought back over our thirty years together—something I'd had plenty of time to do while sitting at her bedside—I remembered times when she'd willingly displayed vulnerability. One episode occurred after the first day of her internship at the Brigham. She had been assigned to the ICU, which was the only possible way to make an already overwhelming experience feel more so. Jane was tough, but even the hardest hard-ass would have floundered after being tossed in the deep end like that.

When she came home on that first evening, she walked straight to the bedroom, sat on the edge of the bed, and started crying.

"I just can't go back," she said between sobs. "It's too much."

"What happened, hon?" I asked, sitting down next to her.

"Too many patients," she said. "And they're so sick. I can't figure out what's wrong with them...."

She looked up at me, pleading.

"I don't know how to take care of them," she said with a hint of a whine.

This was all horrific, of course, but also, as I knew from my own experience, pretty standard stuff. Still, being in the ICU made things that much more intense, and I could see how upsetting it had been.

"Look," I said, "you're exhausted. Why don't you go to sleep? If you wake up tomorrow morning and you still don't want to go back to the hospital, you won't have to. I'll help you find a way out of it."

Jane nodded, lay back in bed, shut her eyes, and went right to sleep with her clothes on.

The next morning, I woke up with her when her alarm rang.

"So," I gingerly asked, "how are you feeling?"

"Don't worry," she said, getting out of bed without looking at me. "I'm going back."

"Okay," I said. "But how are you doing?"

"I'm fine," she said with an edge to her voice. "Absolutely fine. Forget about last night's meltdown."

With that, Jane showered and dressed, and I drove her to work. The window had closed.

I saw no more meltdowns, but there were plenty of times when Jane allowed herself to indulge in displays of tenderness—a different kind of vulnerability. They were all the more special because they were so uncharacteristic. Meant only for me, they had a childlike quality that I found irresistibly endearing.

In year sixteen of our partnership, I finally convinced Jane to abandon the apartment we'd been living in since she was an intern and look for a new place in downtown Boston. The search, which had begun with excited optimism, turned into a death march. Every apartment had at least one flaw—real or imagined—that made Jane reject it. As we slogged our way through the listings, I could see our realtor's growing suspicion that this fussy, acerbic woman wasn't really serious about finding a new home.

Our thousandth showing—at least it felt that way—was a tenth-floor unit overlooking the Charles River. As Jane and I stood at the windows, we realized that the building wasn't located at just any old part of the river—it was at the precise spot where the City of Boston anchors its fireworks barge on the Fourth of July. Jane turned to me and flashed a huge, toothy smile.

"Fireworks," she said softly.

We bought the place. Not because it was a roomy, bright apartment with a perfect layout and a kitchen bigger than almost any you'd find in Back Bay, but because of its unobstructed view of the fireworks.

It didn't disappoint. Every July 4, I'd prepare a faux cookout—stovetop hot dogs, chips, deviled eggs, corn on the cob—and time our dinner to end precisely when the fireworks began. As soon as we heard the Boston Pops start the "1812 Overture," we'd move to the windows and wait for the barrage. In a few minutes, all hell would break loose over the river. The display was transcendent and visceral; we were close enough to feel the percussions in our chest.

But what I loved best was how happy it made Jane. I'd glance at her face, lit up in red or blue or white depending on what was exploding outside, and see a huge smile of delight. No anxieties, no fidgeting, just the pure bliss of a little girl celebrating Independence Day with her family.

Surprisingly, Valentine's Day was another holiday that held meaning for Jane. She gave me a gift every year, but never anything conventional like cards or flowers. Instead, it would be something handmade that had required weeks of planning. One year she constructed a complicated acrostic puzzle with an embedded romantic message. Another year, an arts and crafts project. My favorite was the one she made while I was rehabbing from a training injury by doing "pool running," making jogging-like motions in a swimming pool while supported by floaties around my waist. It was supposed to strengthen my muscles without subjecting them to the pounding of real running. It's great therapy, but it made me look ridiculous. That year, Jane used pipe cleaners to build a detailed model of me in mid-stride and put it in a glass of water. The miniature me carried a sign reading "Happy Valentine's Day." It was a weird, nonsensical gesture, but I loved it.

Big, showy gestures like Valentine's Day presents or my rancid sixtieth birthday cake were rare. More common were small attestations of love, some of which she made to other people. After Jane died, I got a message from one of her particularly devoted trainees. He wanted me to see an email exchange they'd had on the day the Supreme Court struck down the Defense of Marriage Act. He had written to Jane to let her know how happy he was and that he was contemplating marrying his partner. Here's Jane's reply:

I feel honored you'd think of me in this context. Do you know how deeply I care about gay marriage? I think it's because being married to the person I love is the most important thing in the world for me.

And yet, when it came to Jane's relentless expectation to be cared for—to be doted on, to be waited on hand and foot—she was capable of casting aside all considerations of tenderness or sympathy. The prime example was her demand that I devote all of my emotional attention to her and none to my daughter.

Although Anna and I never talked about it, she must have been aware of Jane's disinterest; it was too glaring to ignore. Occasionally, and with great effort, I might be able to drag Jane to a major life event like Anna's high school or college graduation but not much else—no school plays, no birthday parties, no sporting events. And, at whatever gatherings Jane did attend, her body language telegraphed her indifference. A friend of mine once said that, in most social settings, Jane gave the impression that she had somewhere better to be.

The most extreme example of this behavior occurred at Anna's wedding, which took place in the White Mountains of New Hampshire, a three-hour drive north. My mother was well enough to travel then, so she flew from Cleveland to Boston. Jane and I were to pick her up at the airport and take her with us to the wedding.

Jane started our travel day by accusing me of not having provided her with a schedule of the weekend's events and the dress code for each. (Of course, I had.) That meant, according to her, that she had nothing to wear for the rehearsal dinner. How could I be so thoughtless, she kept saying. I'd never seen her so furious.

Jane's foul mood deteriorated with each passing mile. She was barely civil to my mother and disinclined to speak to me. Nothing I said or did could break the spell. I was aware that her unhappiness was driven by her jealousy of Anna and that it would only be exacerbated by watching me walk her down the aisle along with another source of irritation, Anna's mother. Then Jane would have to hear me give speeches about what a wonderful daughter Anna was and how much I loved and admired her. That would be torture.

When we reached the venue, Jane and I went straight to our hotel room. I was hoping that the long drive might have dissipated some of her anger, but I was wrong. As soon as I closed the door, she turned toward me.

"Did you hear what your mother said?" she asked, glaring at me.

"When?" I replied, having no idea what she was talking about.

"In the car. She was talking about your daughter's mother and referred to *her* as your wife."

I snorted a little laugh. Now that she mentioned it, I did remember. My mom had simply made an unfortunate slip of the tongue and I'd thought no more of it.

"There's nothing funny about this," Jane said coolly. "I was sitting right there in the back seat. Your actual wife."

"I know," I said. "It would be thoughtless and insulting coming from anybody else. But my mother is old and has brain damage. If you can't give her a pass, who can you give a pass to?"

"I was right there," she said again, clearly unmollified.

"Yes, you were," I said. "It was a thoughtless mistake and I apologize for her."

I waited a few seconds.

"So," I continued, "can we wash up and join everyone before dinner?"

"I'd sooner drink Drano," Jane said. This was one of her favorite phrases. It told me how mad she still was.

"Come on, hon," I said. "Everyone wants to see you."

"Okay. I'll tell you what," she said, her eyes lighting up. "You want me to pretend that I'm enjoying myself at this fiasco?"

"Well, yes, although it's not a fiasco."

"I'll do it on one condition," she said, ignoring my protest.

"What's that?" I asked. I was willing at this point to do pretty much anything.

"Write my letter for the Austin Prize."

Jane was referring to a prestigious prize that she'd been nominated for by the president of Dana-Farber. There's an odd understanding in the academic world that candidates for these honors are expected to write their own nominating letters, which the nominators lightly edit and then sign. The submission deadline for the Austin Prize was Monday after the wedding, two days away, and true to Jane's procrastinating nature, she hadn't started writing it.

"I'll never forgive you for not telling me about the dress code— or for any of this shit, actually—but I'll participate in the wedding if you write the letter."

"You're kidding, right?" I said.

"I'm dead serious," she replied. "You want me to engage in this horror show that you're responsible for? Write the letter."

Her demand was so bizarre that it was disorienting. One of the secrets of Jane's professional success in a discipline that attracted almost no money or attention was to leverage her meager resources to extract concessions from people in charge. That's what she was doing to me. As horrible as her behavior was, I couldn't help admiring her cunning.

The only way I could ensure a drama-free wedding for Anna was to accede to Jane's request. I spent the next hour crafting a two-page letter that extolled her academic prowess and leadership skills. In exchange, she was civil for the rest of the weekend, although her attitude of "having somewhere better to be" was on full display.

Reader, she won the award.

SIXTEEN

I wish I could say that Jane's near-death experience reset the way we communicated with each other—that we were now more honest and forthright or that we began having heart-to-heart talks about why she had hidden her cancer. But that's not what happened.

Instead, secrecy continued to be Jane's highest priority, and her wish to maintain it went unchallenged. Only Eric and I knew how hard she had worked to keep her cancer hidden and for how long. Her Herculean efforts now had a momentum of their own, one that impelled me to participate in the fiction that her breast cancer had been discovered incidentally—by accident—when she had her pulmonary embolus. This was laughable. It would have been obvious to anyone, but especially to her medically sophisticated colleagues, that the story made no sense.

It didn't matter. No one had the nerve to ask Jane the tough questions that might have forced her to reveal the truth. I understood the reluctance of her colleagues and family members to confront her—Jane could be quite intimidating—and even though difficult questions asked in a caring way might be fair game for close friends, Jane didn't have any.

What I have a harder time understanding is my own disinclination to ask her about her secrecy. This was of a piece with my failure to press Jane about her cancer when she first revealed it on the bathroom floor. Since then, my diffidence had hardened into habit. It, too, seemed to have its own momentum, which made me unwilling to revisit the past and question Jane about her emotional and physical withdrawal. I justified my stance by chiding myself that it was Jane, not me, who was really suffering—she was dying of breast cancer—and it would be unfair to torture her with awkward questions. Yet another of my lame excuses for avoiding an uncomfortable confrontation in favor of letting her dictate the narrative of our marriage.

Instead, something different happened. As the year went on, rather than having heartfelt talks or making tearful confessions, Jane started telling me stories. She would describe events and divulge details that helped explain what, at the time, had been inexplicable behaviors. Mostly, though, she seemed to be using her stories to try to excuse hurtful actions. They were sad and moving tales, but they weren't true apologies and they never fully explained the reasons for her secrecy.

* * *

One morning in November, following the dressing change and Flo's departure, I stayed in Jane's bedroom for a while watching TV with her. After about fifteen minutes, with her eyes fixed on the television screen—not once looking at me—Jane started talking about what had happened to her the last time she traveled.

I pricked up my ears—this was going to be significant. Travel had been an important part of Jane's life for decades until, suddenly and without explanation, it wasn't. She didn't enjoy traveling for its own sake, but she'd been more than willing to take trips for important purposes. Like all academics, she'd spent a lot of time on the road attending meetings or presenting her research findings to her colleagues. But she'd also traveled for personal reasons, one of the most important being to see our friends Michael and Christopher.

We had been devastated when better job opportunities took them to Indianapolis. Happily, we were able to maintain our friendship despite the distance. Although a fundamentally reluctant traveler,

Jane missed Michael and Christopher so much that she was willing to get on an airplane to see them.

Visiting them was hardly a chore. They had purchased an elegant, spacious house that they quickly filled with art. Christopher spent the warm months tending a rambling garden where he grew a variety of beautiful roses. Michael's job—which he performed with aplomb—was to keep the grounds tidy by removing sticks and other debris. Whenever we came to Indy, our hosts would pull out all the stops. It was like staying at the best B&B in the world.

Jane's willingness to visit our friends evaporated suddenly in the early 2000s. As with her other unilateral withdrawals in the years before her collapse, her reasons were utterly opaque. I thought that, of all Jane's social and professional connections, she would have continued to cultivate this one. Michael and Christopher were perplexed but were sensitive enough not to question her.

I also thought that, despite Jane's limited capacity for filial piety, she'd certainly accompany me to my mother's funeral, as she had twenty years earlier to my father's. But I was wrong. My mother had spent the years since my father's death suffering from a horrendous litany of illnesses: heart attack, cardiac arrest, coma and mild brain damage from a lack of oxygen, a stroke that deprived her of vision in one eye, debilitating cardiac chest pains, intestinal damage due to cholesterol blockage of a main artery, repair of an aortic aneurysm, and breast cancer.

True to our father's wishes, my sister and I kept mom in her home throughout her Job-like suffering by making frequent trips to Cleveland to manage her medical and social care. And she survived all of these insults, until she didn't. She died in January 2012, about nine months before Jane's collapse. Jane had not offered to accompany me on my many trips to Cleveland attending to mom's health. That was fine, but I did expect her to come with me to the funeral. I was shocked when Jane said that she couldn't because she had a bad cold. She did not have a bad cold. This hurt me deeply, but Jane made it quite clear that she wasn't going to travel and that she wasn't going to talk about it.

Now, sitting at Jane's bedside, listening to her talk about her last trip out of town, I finally understood why.

She had been invited to give a lecture at Columbia University a few months after my mother's funeral. Although traveling to give talks was a routine part of her job, Jane now revealed that she had been refusing all such requests for a couple of years because she couldn't figure out how to take care of her tumor if she had to be away from home for an extended period. But she had agreed to this one because she figured that she could make it a day trip by train.

Jane started the story by telling me about how she caught the Acela to New York that morning. I held up my hand to stop her.

"Wait," I said. "If you were so concerned about fitting this into a single day, why didn't you fly? Sure, the train could have worked, but maybe the shuttle would have gotten you back and forth faster."

Jane's reply was her first major revelation. Earlier in that year, she had arranged to fly to a meeting, but when she tried to pass through airport security, a TSA agent pulled her aside. He was alarmed by the large mass on the right side of her chest and all of the hardware it contained. In those days, Jane had been secretly dressing her tumor with a jury-rigged concoction of cloth and bandages held together by safety pins. The body scanner had flagged the dressing as an anomaly. Jane tried to explain to the TSA agent that everything on her chest was a medical necessity. He wasn't buying it and led Jane to a private room where she had to undo the dressing and show a female agent what was underneath. Jane was profoundly humiliated and swore she would never fly again.

I was horrified. I took Jane's hand, telling her how sorry I was that this had happened to her. She continued to stare at the TV.

"Now you understand why I couldn't go to your mother's funeral," she said. "I felt bad about not being there with you, but there was just no way I could fly after that experience."

I did understand. The image of Jane undergoing that humiliating, invasive search made me feel sorrier for her than I'd ever felt for anyone.

But...but...what if Jane had confided in me when she first discovered her cancer? I might have convinced her to get medical care and, if that had happened, her doctor might have been able to get her something called a disability notification card from the TSA. I've since learned that these cards may not exempt someone from screening, but when the agents are forewarned, the process can be far more humane. Jane could not have been the only person in America who wanted to get on an airplane with a bulky surgical dressing.

So, as sorry as I was for Jane's humiliation, I was also sorry about all of her—and our—missed opportunities.

She cleared her throat and continued. The day she went to New York, she took the train to Penn Station and caught a cab uptown. She greeted her hosts at Columbia right on time. Her talk went well and she spent another hour or so meeting with colleagues. She then made her excuses, apologizing that she had a train to catch. Her hosts pressed her to stay for dinner—ordinarily an obligation for visiting lecturers—but she was adamant. She had to get home that evening. So, they all said their goodbyes and Jane went down to the street to hail a cab.

As she walked toward a busy intersection, her eyes peeled for a taxi, she was surprised at how out of breath she was. In retrospect, she was quite sick—her breast cancer was getting worse and small blood clots may have already started traveling to her lungs, presaging her huge pulmonary embolus six months later. Spotting a cab, Jane stepped off the curb. But either she misjudged the distance or her legs were weak. Whatever the reason, she fell forward onto the pavement, bruising her hands.

Fortunately, she was more rattled than hurt. A stranger helped her to her feet and into the taxi, which took her to Penn Station.

Jane tried to rally during the cab ride, but as soon as she arrived, she knew she was in trouble. Penn Station is one of the most horrible places on earth. The crowds, the noise, the lights, the smells, being underground—it's Dantesque. Under the best of circumstances, I get completely disoriented whenever I'm there. I couldn't imagine how Jane must have felt. She was weak, short of breath, and had no idea where she was supposed to go to catch her train.

Jane leaned her shoulder against a wall as she made her way toward what she thought was her track, stopping every few minutes to catch her breath. A sympathetic redcap stopped her and asked if she needed help. Although Jane waved him away, he returned a moment later with a wheelchair. The crowds parted as they saw this pale, obviously ill woman being wheeled down the concourse. The redcap got her through the turnstile and onto the train, where she collapsed in her seat. She slept most of the way to Boston and was then able to walk—very slowly—the half-mile from the train station to our apartment.

Jane stopped. I had said I was sorry for her so many times while she'd been talking that the words had lost their meaning. We stared silently at the TV together.

I don't know which image was worse, Jane falling in the street in Upper Manhattan or her nearly collapsing in Penn Station. I couldn't get either one out of my head. In a way, her story was one of remarkable bravery—she had marshaled whatever limited reserves she still had so that she could give her last out-of-town academic lecture, an activity that had been at the heart of her scholarly life. But it was also such a sad story. So much of her suffering had been self-inflicted and, in the end, unnecessary.

Sometimes, though, Jane's tragic tales would remind me of episodes from happier times. One of the few gifts of our last year together was the opportunity it provided to contemplate these moments at length—to hold them like delicate glass figurines and savor their beauty, to use them to displace, at least for a while, the ugliness of our reality. Jane's recounting of her New York disaster had elicited one such memory.

Long before she limited our vacation travel, we used to go on what, for us, were exotic trips every summer. When we were cash-strapped trainees, we would take the ferry to Nantucket and stay in a bed and breakfast. A few years later, when we were flush, we would rent a villa in the Italian countryside for a week. We spent most of our time just hanging out and reading books in the Tuscan sun. For our meals, I would buy fresh ingredients in the nearest town and make us something we both liked.

The villa also served as our base of operations if we wanted to spend an afternoon or evening in a nearby city. There were museums to visit in Florence or architecture to check out in smaller towns like Orvieto. One year we decided to spend a day in Siena. We had heard about the mummified remains of St. Catherine on display in the Basilica of San Domenico and we both knew we had to see them.

The day of our expedition was sunny and blisteringly hot. As we drove to Siena in our rented car, the landscape looked beautiful—like something out of a Renaissance painting—but the heat was oppressive. When we got to the city, I tried to find a place to park close to the church but the best I could manage was a spot fifteen minutes away on foot. We got out of the car and followed a generally downhill route to the church. Once inside, we found our way to the reliquary that housed Catherine's head. It was shaped like a miniature Gothic cathedral with an opening in front, but we couldn't see anything inside. As we leaned dangerously close to get a better look, an annoyed matron dressed in black hissed at us and pointed to the coin box. Apparently, if you fed it ten lire (that's how long ago this was), a light would go on.

We were giddy with anticipation. I fished out a ten-lire coin, inserted it, and stood back. Almost immediately, a small light went on. It illuminated one of the most bizarre things we had ever seen—a small, shrunken head whose eyes were sewn shut. It was missing its nose and its lips were slightly parted in a wry smile. It was wearing a wimple.

We stood and stared with our own mouths agape. Then, after about twenty seconds, the light went out. Jane grabbed my arm and excitedly whispered in my ear, "Do it again!" I found another coin and put it in the slot. The light went on again and we stood rapt. I think we did this four more times before I ran out of change.

We were completely mesmerized by the head of this fourteenth-century woman that had been preserved so lovingly by the church. And not just preserved. Put on display! Maybe if either of us had been Catholic we would have been less gobsmacked. But, being heathens, we felt like anthropologists who had stumbled upon the exotic rites of a lost civilization.

We walked out of the church and into the sunlight, highly pleased with ourselves. As we headed back to the car, we continued our animated talk about Catherine's head and what it all meant. Suddenly, Jane stopped. She took a step into the street and sat down on the curb.

"I can't go any farther," she said, looking up at me.

The downhill path to the church had become an uphill path to the car, and the combination of the heat plus Jane's constitutional weakness had undone her.

I told her that we were, at most, only ten minutes away from the car. No dice. I said that I didn't know for sure that I'd be able to find her once I got the car. (It's amazing how irrelevant this story would be if it had happened in the era of cell phones and GPS.) Jane said she didn't care. She trusted that I'd do my best and she was willing to take the chance that she'd be lost forever.

I walked to the car, shaking my head. I did have trouble retracing my route back to Jane on those twisty, one-way streets. But I eventually found her, and we drove together back to the villa.

* * *

A television commercial for a personal injury lawyer screaming at the top of his lungs brought me back to the present. I wasn't in Italy anymore. In fact, I wouldn't ever be with Jane in Italy or anywhere else fun, exotic, or just pleasant. That was all over.

SEVENTEEN

For eight months, Eric's treatments would slow the growth of Jane's cancer, keeping it at bay. While her nearly imperceptible decline was a blessing, it nurtured Jane's unrealistic hopes of returning to her professional life. But the cancer wasn't shrinking, and its presence in so many organs—lungs, liver, bones, skin—continued to make her weak. Every attempt to reengage at work ended in disappointment.

One of the most heart-rending was her decision to attend an award ceremony honoring her achievements as a mentor. About a year prior to her collapse, I'd worked with Dana-Farber's philanthropy department to persuade a donor to endow a yearly prize for outstanding mentorship. It would recognize a faculty member with a noteworthy record of supporting the careers of students, fellows, and younger faculty. Jane was a top candidate long before anyone knew about her cancer.

In fact, Jane's reputation as a role model and mentor extended far beyond the Farber. She was famous for inspiring intense personal loyalty in nearly everyone who worked with her, from young trainees to peers. She'd cultivated this status in a variety of settings but nowhere more effectively than at the annual meetings of the American Society for Clinical Oncology, or ASCO.

More than forty thousand oncologists from around the world attend this combination trade show and scientific conference. It's a zoo. While important advances in the treatment of cancer are discussed there, it's also an opportunity for pharmaceutical companies to peddle their wares to the doctors who might prescribe them. The first thing attendees see when they walk into the convention center is an acre of elaborately outfitted booths manned by attractive young people handing out swag.

In Jane's heyday, oncology was dominated by a handful of companies that charged high prices for marginally effective drugs. This was, of course, a serious problem, but Jane's group at Dana-Farber had the authority and skill to tackle it—her faculty were experts in health services research, a discipline that examines the utilization, quality, cost, and impact of medical interventions and governmental policies. They and like-minded scientists published a slew of high-profile studies questioning the cost-effectiveness of expensive cancer drugs. Not surprisingly, their analyses placed them squarely outside the ASCO mainstream.

Jane cleverly turned their outcast status to her advantage. While other oncologists were presenting the results of drug company–funded clinical trials to audiences of thousands in the main lecture hall, the health services researchers, who numbered only a few hundred, would meet in a small room next door. Jane's strategy was to make a sincere and highly visible show of taking seriously all the presentations that were being made in that diminutive venue. She'd listen carefully to every lecturer—from grad students to tenured professors—and when they were done, she'd slowly make her way to the microphone and offer a killer comment.

Sometimes, she'd begin by saying, "Isn't the point of this study really..." and go on to help the speaker reframe the presentation in a way that made it better.

Other times, if the study had been done poorly, she'd provide a brief, cogent critique. Usually, she'd be kind. But if the presenter was a pompous know-it-all who'd made fundamental analytic errors, she'd flay him. The tiny crowd ate it up.

Jane's skillful support of good speakers, and her deliberate contrast of the scholarly activity in the health services room with the rock concert in the main hall, meant that the field coalesced around her. When the presentations were over, she would consolidate her status by suggesting that the twenty or so leading lights, plus a few trainees, all go out to dinner together. Even as the drug companies were hosting their fancy evening receptions—also known as "Infinite Shrimp"—Jane and her colleagues found funky Thai restaurants that could accommodate their small crowd. They ate family style with Jane presiding as mother.

Jane had also been an exceptional mentor closer to home—not only for talented trainees like Deb but for others whose promise as medical researchers might not have been so obvious. Some young doctors complete their training only to decide, perhaps inaccurately, that they're ill-suited for the research career they thought they wanted. One starts thinking that her skills might be a better fit for writing poetry than pursuing science; another's stutter makes him shrink from taking the aggressive stance needed to establish an academic career; a third may be brilliant but her autism spectrum disorder has so far kept her from receiving academic recognition.

Jane's gift was to see the talent and promise in these individuals. She created a home for them in her division—she lovingly referred to it as The Island of Misfit Toys—and worked closely with each one to craft a successful career. A great mentor can divine someone's skills and match that person to the kind of work that best exploits those skills. That's what Jane did for the young physicians and scientists who came through her division. And that's why they'd take a bullet for her.

It was no surprise, then, that the selection committee for the mentorship award chose Jane as its first recipient. To celebrate her achievement, the Farber's event planners hoped to hold a ceremony in late January. Jane had just started toying with the idea of going back to work, at least for a few days a week, so she thought that attending the event in person might be a good test of her stamina.

But there were lots of reasons to doubt the feasibility of her plan—she'd have to deal with the tumor mass on her chest with its bulky surgical dressing, her shortness of breath which necessitated supplemental oxygen, her painful bone metastases. Most debilitating, though, was a general weakness caused largely by a complication of her cancer known as cachexia, an unrelenting loss of muscle mass that cannot be reversed by increasing food intake. Mercifully, in Jane's case, it hadn't affected her face. From the neck up she looked just about the same as she always had. But the rest of her body was wasting away.

Jane was acutely aware of these physical changes and confided in Flo one morning that she might be too self-conscious about her muscle loss to be seen in public. Flo swung into action. Naturally, being Flo, she knew all there was to know about padded underwear and so, from a company called Bubbles Bodywear, she ordered foam and silicone "butt pads" that fit into Jane's underwear. When the package from Bubbles arrived, Flo stayed for an extra hour to help Jane figure out how to use the pads. Then she had Jane give me a fashion show so I could see how great they made her look in her clothes. It was all hilarious in its own sad way.

Ultimately, Jane couldn't bring herself to use the Bubbles. But she did let Flo help her select an outfit and do some tailoring that partially hid Jane's weight loss. Then Flo artfully manipulated the silicone cutlets on the left side of Jane's chest to balance the tumor dressing on the right.

The last bit of preparation for the award ceremony involved her hair. Jane had gone gray in her thirties and had been coloring it ever since, but she was so half-hearted about the process that she only did touch-ups twice a year. Although her visits to the salon were infrequent, they were eagerly anticipated by the people who worked there. She would spend hours entertaining them with stories, anecdotes, insights—her usual repertoire of fun stuff. From the stylist to the hair-washer to the receptionist to the person who swept the floor, they all loved it when she showed up.

The salon's owner, another fan, was eager to help when I asked if he could arrange an appointment for Jane to get her hair colored at a time when the place might be relatively empty. She was still very self-conscious about her illness and didn't even want strangers to think there was anything wrong with her. He obligingly cleared the salon's schedule for a few hours on a Tuesday afternoon so that Jane could be alone.

On the appointed day, I helped her dress and then, with my arm around her waist, we left the apartment and made our way to the car. We left her oxygen behind to see how she'd do without it for a few hours. I gently lowered Jane into the passenger seat and drove the quarter mile to the salon, pulling up as close as I could to the entrance. An elevator brought us up to the second floor and when the doors opened, everyone rushed to greet Jane, to talk to her, and to guide her to a chair. The receptionist, a talented artist who we had known for years—I got my hair cut at the same place—had gifts for Jane. She gave her a tiara and a feather boa, which Jane modeled with aplomb. I hung around while she got her hair done and worked the crowd.

Coming home after her appointment was a struggle. I think Jane was surprised at how thoroughly the excursion had depleted her. But she was undaunted—she was determined to attend the award ceremony in person and without an oxygen tank at her side.

On the appointed day, I helped Jane get ready the same way I had for her salon visit. And, just like that day, she was mobbed by her fans when she entered the room. Jane clearly enjoyed the attention, but I could feel her sag as she was leaning on my shoulder so I made excuses and guided her to a chair in the front row.

The program had been organized by Deb, Jane's first trainee and designated successor as division chief. To start the ceremony, she gave a slide presentation describing, among other things, the twenty or so individuals Jane had trained who went on to become research leaders in their own rights. Several now held prestigious academic positions. They had sent Deb their thoughts about Jane and, after spending some time talking about her own interactions with Jane, she wrapped up by quoting from a few of them:

> *"Jane is like a third parent. Precisely when our parents don't have a clue how to help us through the most pressing academic challenges, Jane steps in to serve that role."*

> *"Every time I left Jane's office, I felt inspired in a way that I feel at almost no other time. She has this knack for making you feel like your work is important, your personal life is important, and you are important."*

> *"Meeting with Jane on a regular basis was truly one of the highlights of my job. When she put her feet up on the desk and popped a piece of gum into her mouth, I knew I had her full attention."*

Then it was time for Jane to speak. I helped her to the podium, but she was too weak to stand so someone brought a chair to the front of the room. I gently lowered Jane into it and returned to my own seat. Jane spoke from her heart for about five minutes. She talked about how much the mentorship award meant to her but, even more, how much all of her trainees had meant to her. It was a lovely speech. There wasn't a dry eye in the house.

In the car, on our way home, I told Jane that I thought it had been a wonderful event and that her remarks were right on target.

"Yeah," she replied. "I guess so. But it felt like a funeral."

I understood what she meant and tried to argue a little, pointing out that everyone would have said exactly the same things even if she had been perfectly healthy. She just nodded. She was discouraged because she had made a superhuman effort just to attend an hour-long ceremony that left her exhausted. She was now forced to face the fact that her plan to return to work, even for two days a week, was not realistic.

Another loss. So much had been taken away from Jane this year—her health, her autonomy, her future. One of the few remaining vestiges of her old life was her title as chief of the Division of Population Sciences at the Farber. I wasn't surprised that she clung to it despite mounting evidence that she could no longer do the job.

Jane was only the second chief in the division's history—she had succeeded its founder—and one of the few women at the Institute to hold such an elevated academic leadership position. She'd been a great division chief. In her eleven years at the helm, she had hired several outstanding faculty members and attracted impressive amounts of research funding. Her division developed an international reputation for being at the forefront of cancer outcomes measurements and health policy research.

A vital component of leadership roles like these is modeling academic success for the other faculty in the division. Jane had done this superbly. Even after her pulmonary embolus, her research stayed on track partly because of its inherent momentum and partly because her colleagues took up some of the slack. Amazingly, she continued to publish high-profile papers from bed.

But another component of a chief's responsibilities—the one that differentiates a leader from an ordinary faculty member—is the business of running an academic division: things like hiring new faculty, fighting the hospital administration for resources, and developing division-wide strategies for the future. Jane loved this aspect of the job and had been good at it. She was particularly adept at guiding her junior faculty through the thickets of the promotion process. I benefitted from that skill, too, whenever Jane gave me advice about my own academic advancement.

Now, though, she was having a hard time attending to these duties and, after several months of relative neglect, the division was feeling rudderless. To be fair, Jane tried to be diligent about answering her email when she was feeling up to it and participated in conference calls about division issues when she had the strength. But these were no substitute for the effect that a leader's physical presence can have on an organization.

Then there's the informational value you can only glean from face-to-face interactions. Only during in-person meetings do you detect the subtle eyeroll of a passive-aggressive colleague who's obstructing progress. Only in meetings do you appreciate the hesitant body language of a shy mid-level worker who, with a little encouragement, could become a key contributor. In those pre-Zoom days, Jane couldn't make these kinds of on-the-spot assessments from home.

In the absence of in-person management, conflicts began to arise in the division that tapped into old grudges and misunderstandings. Because of the dominance of molecular biology and genetics in cancer research, Jane believed that Dana-Farber's leadership neither understood nor valued the kind of science that had made her and her division famous. As evidence, she would trot out a story from early in her career when she had been asked to give a talk about her research to the Institute's trustees. The president of Dana-Farber at the time, a Nobel Prize–winning basic scientist, was also in the audience and, after her presentation, asked her incredulously, "Do you mean you can actually get this kind of work published?" She cited this as proof that leadership knew nothing about what she and her colleagues were doing.

"That was twenty years ago," I said to her the last time she'd brought this up. "You do understand that everything's changed now, don't you?"

"Nothing's changed," she snorted. "Genetics is the only thing anyone cares about. That and maybe testing new drugs so that people can make money."

"You can't take that attitude with me anymore," I said. "I know better. You forget that I've seen firsthand the largesse you've received from the Institute."

"Oh, please," she said, waving her hand dismissively. "They've given us so much less than they've given everyone else."

I was very familiar with Jane's "us-versus-them" move, the one that had made her colleagues love her at ASCO. It had worked just as well at the Farber, where she'd used it to rally her faculty around her and win their loyalty. They saw Jane as their protector—a tireless advocate who would go to any lengths to secure the resources and respect they felt entitled to.

The fact was that Jane had succeeded. She'd gotten most of what she'd asked for from the Farber, so I was not going to let her get away with playing the victim. At least not with me.

"First of all," I said, "your division is one of the centerpieces of the huge grant that supports the cancer center."

"Oh, that's just because the National Cancer Institute makes Dana-Farber do that."

"Second," I continued, "I've seen the amount of money the Institute has given you to recruit faculty. Your recruiting has outpaced most of the other divisions."

Silence.

"Third, and most important," I said, "you know that, in the administrative world, nothing says love like research space. The Institute just gave your division two full floors of prime real estate and spent a ton of money renovating it. For Christ's sake, they even put a two-story atrium in the kitchen area for you."

As I spoke, Jane began to smile, proud of the tangible assets she'd wrested from the institution. I was smiling too. I had to admit that she was a good division chief.

But we'd had that conversation over a year ago. By late spring, with her condition deteriorating, she no longer had the wherewithal to fight for her division. She couldn't muster the stamina for the in-person interactions that forceful advocacy requires.

As a result, institutional leadership was worried. Back when Jane first came home from the hospital after her pulmonary embolus, her boss, the chair of the Department of Medical Oncology, had granted her request that she be allowed to continue as division chief as long as her cancer wasn't progressing. But that understanding had been reached in the early fall when everyone assumed that she'd eventually be well enough to come back to work. Now it was clear that, because of Jane's weakness, she wouldn't be able to return and the chair was concerned about the impact her prolonged absence was having on the division and its faculty. So, he'd started canvassing the senior members of the division about their needs.

Unfortunately, he initiated those discussions without talking to Jane first. Big mistake. Deb was one of the senior faculty the chair had talked to first and, of course, she loyally told Jane what was happening.

"I can't believe this," Jane said to me after talking to Deb. "He's going behind my back, stirring up the faculty so he can force me out of my chief position."

She looked off into space for a moment.

"I know what's really going on here," she continued, shaking her head. "I'm not stupid. He's taking advantage of my illness—which, by the way, is *cancer* for god's sake. Does that mean nothing to a cancer institute? He's using my illness as an excuse to replace me with someone who would move the division's science closer to molecular biology and genetics. Which just happens to be what he's interested in."

The chair had, in fact, talked to some of the faculty about their interests in these areas but only to try to understand where they wanted to see their division's future science go. But Jane saw those conversations as a direct challenge to her non-molecular, non-genetic research interests, the foundation on which she had built her division.

She was as angry and disappointed as I had ever seen her. A few months earlier, she had modified her will to create an endowment at Dana-Farber for the support of rising young faculty in Population

Sciences—her academic children. She was now threatening to withdraw her bequest.

"It breaks my heart," she said, "that the institute I've given my life to would let this happen to me."

It broke my heart too. She really had devoted her life to Dana-Farber. But the hard fact was that she hadn't been well enough to meet with people in her division for months, and the wonderful academic enterprise she'd built was suffering.

I knew how important being division chief was to Jane. So many of the things that gave her life meaning—having an impact on disease, influencing clinical practice, mentoring young professionals—were made possible by her leadership role. Giving it up would be a wrenching loss, but it would also be an explicit admission that she was dying. I understood why she was lashing out and accusing her boss of underhanded behavior—she was facing a horrible truth that, until now, she had been able to sidestep. No wonder her response was, "How could they do this to me?"

But over the next few weeks, as Jane continued to stew, she also became physically weaker. Eventually, she admitted to herself that she could no longer lead her division.

"All right," she said to me one afternoon, "I'm throwing in the towel."

"What are you talking about?" I asked.

"I admit it. They're right," she said. "I can't run PopSci anymore. Let Deb do it."

She seemed more angry than sad.

"Are you sure?"

"Positive," she said. "Would you do me a favor and write an announcement that I'm stepping down? I can give it to Deb to send out in a blast email."

This again. It was a sadder and less farcical echo of the recommendation letter she forced me to write at Anna's wedding. I chose not to point that out.

"Of course," I said. "I'm so sorry about this, hon."

"Can't be helped," she said.

I wrote a draft describing the leadership change. It said that Deb would take over as chief and try to continue Jane's visionary work.

Deb and I spoke after I sent her the announcement.

"This is so sad," she said.

"It is," I agreed. "It sounds like an obituary. But it's also necessary."

"Yes, it is," she said. "It really is. Things are a little chaotic here and this will provide some clarity."

Deb paused.

"Tell Jane that I will run everything by her," she continued. "The decisions about recruitment and promotion, the grants, the papers, everything. Does that make sense?"

"Yes, it does," I said. "That will make her happy."

"This will be Jane's division for as long as she's alive."

EIGHTEEN

Jane brought the same unwavering focus on controlling the narrative of her career to dictating the terms of our marriage. Although she ended up firmly in the driver's seat, that's not how things had started. We'd begun as equals, sensitive about the obligations that new couples impose on each other. But when the balance of power started tilting toward Jane, the change was so gradual that I wasn't conscious of it or, if I was, I would rationalize my way into accepting it. During our first year, I looked up one day to find that we were spending all our time at her apartment instead of mine—that was okay, I guess. Later, when we were living together, I was doing all of the household chores—well, she was an intern, what did I expect? Then she refused to have anything to do with Anna. Maybe that one wasn't so easy to elide but, by now, I was in too deep.

I might have pushed back but...but I didn't want to—or, more accurately, I was convinced that I couldn't. I thought that by making the concessions Jane sought early in the relationship, I could tie her to me. But then, as time went on and her demands increased, I felt trapped. I'd established a pattern of behavior that Jane had come to expect and, frankly, exploit. I didn't think I could flout her expectations without jeopardizing the marriage.

And I did not want to do that. I'd already been through one failed marriage with Anna's mother. I had a sense, *pace* Oscar Wilde, that to fail in one marriage may be regarded as a misfortune; to fail in two before age forty looks like carelessness—or worse, a character defect. I needed this marriage to succeed.

* * *

Some of Jane's demands were innocent enough and even had a bit of sweetness, like her refusal to give up my grandmother's wedding ring. But even the issue of wedding rings was tainted by her need for control.

After our Nantucket wedding, Jane started asking whether I might consider wearing a wedding ring now that we were officially married. My father had never worn a ring, nor had most of my male relatives, nor had I during my first marriage. Jane knew that history and, until now, hadn't expressed any discomfort about my ringless state. But I respected her wishes and if she wanted her husband to wear a wedding ring, I would give it a try.

So, one Saturday afternoon we made an excursion to Boston's tiny diamond district. We must have visited at least seven stores—each was a hole in the wall fronting a vast hidden selection—and at every stop I tried on a dozen rings. Jane was an intense shopper. No matter what she might be looking for, she had to be satisfied that she had seen all available options before she would allow herself to make a decision. Choosing a vacation rental was sheer torture. She had to review every home within a fifty-mile radius, including many that were clearly unacceptable, before she invariably chose the first one we had looked at.

I thought that our forced march through Boston's jewelry stores was just another example of Jane's completeness fetish. I was wrong. At the seventh store, midway through my modeling its selection of men's wedding rings, Jane put up her hand.

"Stop. Take it off. We're done," she said.

"Why? You must have liked at least one of the rings we've seen," I said.

"That's not it. Every time you put on a ring, you look henpecked. Don't wear a wedding ring. Forget I ever said anything."

Her reversal was not as surprising as it seemed; I knew what she was worried about. When we first started dating, Jane would vacillate wildly between her certainty that we were meant for each other—as in her early prediction that we'd get married—and her fear that I wasn't worthy of her. Her big concern was that I might be weak in some unspecified manner. For the first few months we were together, she would say, "I can't stand wimpy men. You're not a wimp, are you?" She seemed to be worried about how she'd be perceived—that she herself might be seen as weak if she were in a relationship with a weak man.

Now, years later, she was still bouncing between being pleased with a man who would do her bidding and her fear that an overly compliant partner would appear to be "henpecked." But either way, Jane was the one calling the shots—she had given up on the ring because *she* didn't want me to wear it, not because I didn't.

I'll admit that, by not asking her to consider my wishes, I let Jane commandeer the wedding ring question. Although not particularly happy about rolling over so readily, I did it in this situation and countless others to keep the peace. There were times, though, when I was inclined to yield to her because I thought that doing so would actually benefit me. It seemed the best course, for example, when Jane tried to mold my career—she had been so adept at advancing her own that it seemed foolish not to heed her advice for mine.

But dig a little deeper and here, too, her motives were not purely altruistic. Jane had always been sensitive about the professional status of her partners and was attracted to men who outranked her—a superior at the think tank in Washington, a professor at her medical school, and me, a senior resident at her training hospital. The appeal was entirely self-referential—Jane wanted her partner to have sufficient standing to reflect well on her.

During our early years together, Jane was satisfied because I occupied a higher place in the academic hierarchy than she did. But her raw talent soon turbo-charged her climb up the ladder, and by the early 2000s she had zoomed past me—she had become a full professor with tenure while I languished at a lower rank. The inversion of our professional positions didn't bother me very much, not even when my misguided department chair took me aside after Jane's promotion to ask if I'd be troubled by the fact that my wife would now be making a higher salary than me. Mind? I thought it was fantastic!

But the change seemed to bother Jane. Although my career was still advancing—albeit more slowly than hers—and I was likely to be promoted in a few years, she brooded about the disparity in our trajectories. That's why she was so interested when I told her about a newly created executive position, chief scientific officer, designed to oversee the research program at Dana-Farber. Our CEO had offered me the job but I was unsure about accepting because, if I did, I would have to reduce the amount of time I could spend on my laboratory research. Even though my academic progress had been sluggish, at least I understood the rules for getting promoted to professor. I had no idea what the professional rules would be for a CSO.

But Jane was curiously certain about this new opportunity.

"What are you going to do about this CSO job?" she asked one Sunday afternoon as we drove back to Boston from a wedding of one of her trainees in Rhode Island.

"Honestly, I don't know yet," I said.

"Really? Everything you've told me makes it seem like an ideal job for you. Isn't that what David said too?"

She was referring to a past president of Dana-Farber, who had called me into his office a few weeks earlier to urge me to take the job.

"Yeah, he did," I said. "David does have an impressive track record of placing the right people in the right positions. I suppose I ought to listen to him."

"I suppose you ought to. He's right."

"I don't know. In my world, only failed scientists become administrators. I wonder if that's what David was really telling me."

"What, that you're a failed scientist?"

"Yes, exactly."

"Did he actually say that?"

"No, but I'm not sure he'd be that direct."

"Really?" Jane asked, shaking her head and smiling. "David's a pretty direct guy. He never had any trouble refusing my requests for Institute resources. If he thought you were a failed scientist, he would have said so."

"I guess," I admitted.

"Instead," she barreled ahead, "he's telling you that you're the perfect person for this new job. I think he's right."

"Do you, now?" I said. "What do you actually know about the CSO job?"

"Only what you've told me, I'll admit. But the job does seem to align with your skills. You're good with people, you see the big picture, you're highly organized. Plus, you'd have a seat at the small table where big decisions get made. You'd have real clout."

There it was. I don't doubt that Jane was sincere in her assessment of how my skills might serve me as CSO, but she also liked the fact that taking the job would make me an executive. From her point of view—not mine—becoming a member of the vaunted C-suite would restore the balance of power in our marriage. It would give me a status worthy of her own. Plus, I'd still be on the academic track and likely to be promoted in a few years.

As it happened, Jane was right; the job was a perfect fit. I was good at bringing groups together to advance Dana-Farber's research, and I liked strategizing with other leaders about the future of that research. But there was a dark side. The position was a target for every narcissistic faculty member who felt entitled to more space and more money than they were currently allotted. An ever-expanding chunk of my time was spent finding gentle—and occasionally not so gentle—ways of saying no. This was an unwelcome development for someone fundamentally averse to conflict like me. Plus, Jane later tried to use her influence on me to get more resources for the projects she was interested in. I might have been the only person who was surprised by her boldness.

Because I was the Institute's first CSO, I was inventing the job on the fly, always unsure about where it was heading. I could never be certain that the next challenge might not defeat me, and I had a nagging suspicion that winding down my lab research in favor of administrative work might turn out to be an irreversible step. I had no Plan B if the CSO job blew up.

Despite my concerns, I threw myself into the work. It was inherently interesting, as advertised, but the focused intensity and long hours I devoted to it were also about something else: an escape from an increasingly painful life at home.

* * *

As we entered our third decade together, Jane's demands and odd proclivities became much more difficult to live with. What had started as a quirky, endearing neediness in someone otherwise so hypercompetent had evolved into a collection of worrisome behaviors that had troubling implications. I can see now that they were driven by her cancer, both her fear of it and her obsessive need to keep it a secret. But at the time, they seemed inexplicable.

To keep our partnership on an even keel, I had figured out ways to accommodate Jane's expanding needs and idiosyncrasies. Things became much more difficult when she soured on sex. I had always felt lucky that the sexual excitement we'd experienced when we were a new couple had barely faded over our first twenty years together. Then suddenly, in the early 2000s, something shifted. Jane started avoiding any physical contact with me and rebuffed all my advances. After decades of sleeping together in the nude, she suddenly appeared one night in a floor-length caftan that zipped up to her chin. The message could not have been clearer.

I was unhappy and confused and wanted to talk to her about what had changed.

"Hon," I began one cloudless afternoon while we were having lunch on the patio of our rented villa in the Caribbean, "can we talk about sex?"

No response. Jane stared straight ahead, seemingly absorbed in the picture-perfect ocean view.

"Really?" I asked. "No comment?"

"What do you want me to say?" she replied, finally turning toward me with an angry look.

"I don't have anything I specifically want you to say."

"Well, then, what *do* you want?" she said, refocusing her attention on a sailboat luffing in the distance.

I waited to see if Jane would answer her own question. When she didn't, I continued.

"I want to know why we haven't touched each other in a year. I want to know what I did to repulse you so thoroughly."

Jane kept staring straight ahead.

"Look, I love you," I said. "And I think you love me. I want to know why you decided that part of our lives is over."

Finally, Jane turned to look at me. Tears were rolling down her cheeks. She started to speak but sobbed instead.

"I'm sorry," she said. "I'm sorry.... I can't talk about it."

"Hon," I said, reaching for her hand, "you can and I'll listen."

"No," she nearly screamed, pulling her hand back. "I can't ever talk about it and neither can you."

She shot up from the table and walked quickly into the villa. I watched her slam the bedroom door behind her.

I stayed on the patio. I had finally worked up the courage to talk to her and got nothing for the effort.

A few hours later, Jane was back on the patio, acting as if nothing had happened. She took a swim in the pool and asked me about our dinner plans. It was clear that she'd never agree to talk about sex. So, faced with her intransigence, I had to figure out whether I could accept this new reality and stay in the marriage. I thought about it when we got home and eventually came to the conclusion that I was still in love with her and happy with essentially every other aspect of our lives. I sensed—or, perhaps, hoped—that her aversion to sex, like her addiction to computer games, was not an aversion to me. Maybe I was fooling myself, I thought, but the abruptness of the change and the absence of any other indication that she found me repulsive made it seem as if this whole business were about something else, although I still had no idea what that "something" might be. Regardless, my decision gave me yet another way to avoid further confrontation.

Things didn't improve. In fact, a year or two later, we stopped sleeping in the same bed. The reasons were complicated. For Jane to fall asleep at night, she had to have the television on. She said that listening to TV distracted her from her thoughts—the same way, I assume, that computer games did. I, in contrast, am highly sensitive to sound and cannot fall asleep unless I'm swaddled in silence. So, sleeping together had always involved accommodation.

Every night, I'd lie next to Jane and watch TV until I heard the sound of regular breathing from her side of the bed—an indication, I hoped, that she had fallen asleep. I would reach gingerly for the remote and turn off the television. One of two things would happen next. Either there would be silence, allowing me to fall asleep too, or Jane would say, "Not yet," in which case I would have to turn the TV back on and start the whole process again. I tried earplugs, of course, but no brand, not even custom-fitted, could block the sound of the TV.

This was another compromise I was willing to make, one that I had made for two decades; I have seen every *Law & Order* episode at least ten times. But right around the time that Jane turned from sex, her need for TV sharply increased. Now there were nights she couldn't fall asleep at all, which meant that the TV was on until dawn. At first this would only happen intermittently and, when it did, I would retreat to the guest bedroom. Eventually, though, as Jane's need for distraction became more intense, I just gave up and the guest room became my permanent bedroom. Again, no discussion—just another ratcheting down in intimacy.

* * *

If anyone had asked how I was doing around that time, I would have answered, "Just fine," and I would have believed what I was saying. I was performing capably in a meaningful job that I liked well enough, and I was in a stable, long-term marriage. But, in fact, I was suffering. More specifically, I felt trapped, imprisoned by circumstances that seemed to deteriorate with every passing year.

Things got much worse after Jane's bleeding episode on the bathroom floor. That's when I started having suicidal thoughts. I'm fairly sure that I wouldn't have acted on them, but they were very concrete and their content was always the same: my plan was to jump from our tenth-floor apartment. In my fantasies, I would always choose the same window, the one farthest to the right in Jane's bedroom. I pictured myself walking up to it, raising the sash, lifting the screen out of the way, climbing onto the sill, leaning out, and pushing off. Sometimes, I'd add little details like checking to make sure I dove headfirst to increase the odds that I'd kill myself rather than just break a bunch of bones.

I had enough insight to take this as a sign that I could use some counseling. I'd undergone analysis during medical school and knew how beneficial talking to a psychiatrist could be. But I didn't seek help now, because if I did, I would have to tell the shrink about Jane's secrets and I could not bring myself to betray her to a stranger, even one bound by confidentiality.

Despite their violence, my fantasies of suicide were oddly calming. The possibility of an escape from my misery—even via a mechanism as gruesome as defenestration—was a balm. I would replay my scenario two or three times a week, often to help me fall asleep at night.

Life with Jane was not the sole cause of my suicidal ideation. My job, as much as I liked it, had become difficult and exasperating, and, again, I wasn't sure where the intense effort it required was leading.

So, I was feeling trapped both by my work and by my marriage. No wonder, then, that I fantasized about taking a way out. After Jane's stay in the ICU, though, my thoughts of suicide vanished. I had become too engrossed in the day-to-day mechanics of caring for her to indulge them. In retrospect, I'm frightened for my old self. I was profoundly miserable and had convinced myself that I had nowhere to turn for help. There was no guarantee that I'd find a way out.

NINETEEN

M y claustrophobic perception of having no control over my life
grew more acute when Jane came home from the hospital
after her pulmonary embolus. My existence was now utterly ruled by
the rhythms of caring for her cancer and its complications. Although
my feelings about this burden might have been understandable, I
was embarrassed by my unhappiness: my problems were nothing
compared with hers—Jane had metastatic breast cancer and it was
going to kill her.

Despite that grim knowledge, we were able to lull ourselves into
a sort of complacency for a few months. The treatments Eric prescribed were making Jane feel a little better. During the fall she had
regained some strength and at times felt good enough to talk about
returning to work. We all—me, Jane, Eric, Flo, Olivia—tacitly agreed
to pretend that she had a future.

By mid-winter, though, signs of her advancing cancer couldn't
be ignored. From then on, Jane was subjected to cycles of hopeful
expectations followed by crashing disappointments, the first one
involving the tumor on her chest. It would be impossible to over-
state the impact of this enormous, rotting, bleeding mass—and the
daily dressing changes it demanded—on Jane's quality of life. She
couldn't indulge in fantasies of returning to work if that thing were
still there. She wanted to have it surgically removed.

Eric thought that Jane would never be in better shape to tolerate
surgery than she was in late January and early February, so he asked

Sue the surgeon for her opinion. She said that an operation might be feasible, but it would be a big, complicated procedure. In addition to the mass itself, she would have to remove the underlying muscle and ribs to which the tumor was attached. Then, while Jane was still under anesthesia, a plastic surgeon would try to cover the huge open chest wound with skin grafts harvested from her buttocks and thighs. It would be a risky surgery followed by a prolonged recovery.

We all knew that as much as removing the mass might improve Jane's quality of life, it would have no effect on the cancer that had already spread to her liver, lungs, and bones. Those were the tumor deposits that would eventually kill her. So, the question we had to ask ourselves was why would we subject someone to such a mammoth operation knowing that it would not prolong that person's life? Jane understood the implications of this question well—probably better than anyone—but still wanted to pursue the possibility.

But before surgery could even be considered, a very practical problem had to be addressed. Given the cancer in Jane's lungs and her chronic shortness of breath, Sue was concerned about whether Jane could survive prolonged general anesthesia. So, Sue asked an anesthesiologist colleague to evaluate her. The anesthesiologist was very sympathetic but worried about Jane's continued shortness of breath, so she recommended that she have another CT-angiogram to make sure that there were no new clots in her lungs.

A few days later, I bundled Jane back into our car and took her to the hospital for the test. Fortunately, the CT-angiogram showed no clots. However, it did show that her chest mass had grown since the fall, as had her lymph nodes and the tumor deposits in her lungs. Her cancer was advancing despite Eric's treatments.

On sober reassessment, Sue was now reluctant to undertake such an enormous operation for a benefit that, although real, was vanishingly small. The extensive skin grafting would require frequent dressing changes, perhaps continuing for months. Jane would be trading her current misery for a future that sounded just as bad.

Reluctantly, Jane agreed that surgery was impractical. The escape hatch that she'd been eyeing so hopefully had slammed shut. She was stuck in her torture chamber.

It was now painfully clear that Eric's treatments had stopped working. Jane's tumors were getting bigger and she was feeling worse. She continued to refuse traditional chemotherapy, so the question was what to try next.

When Jane first decided to treat herself in secret, she had guessed that her breast cancer was the kind in which tumor growth is stimulated by female sex hormones like estrogen. She was playing the odds—that's the most common type of breast cancer in women of her age. So, she had started taking tamoxifen, an oral inhibitor of the estrogen receptor, the molecule in breast cancer cells through which estrogen works. In fact, Jane now said that she had seen some tumor shrinkage when she first started taking the drug but the effect had worn off after a year.

Jane's experiment told Eric that her cancer was, at least partly, driven by hormones working through the estrogen receptor. He was not surprised to hear that her cancer had eventually become resistant to tamoxifen, which is a common enough occurrence. Fortunately, he had a backup plan: a more potent antiestrogen, ful-vestrant, which works on breast cancers that become resistant to tamoxifen. The problem was that it had to be given by injection and our visiting nurses, Flo and Olivia, weren't allowed to administer it. That meant going to the hospital.

Jane was intensely anxious about getting her treatment at Dana-Farber. She was still fixated on keeping her medical condition a secret and was afraid that she might run into someone she knew, which would lead to pitying looks and uncomfortable questions. But Eric and the nursing staff were keyed into her concern and promised that they would do whatever they could to make her visit a stealthy one. Jane was convinced but wary.

When the day came for her injection, I helped her into her wheelchair, took her down to the car, and maneuvered her into the passenger seat. We drove to the valet parking entrance at the hospital, where I transferred her to another wheelchair. From there, we meandered through back hallways and service elevators up to the breast cancer clinic. The last elevator deposited us just a few feet from a treatment room that had been specifically prepared for Jane. I hustled her in and we high-fived because no one had seen us.

In the treatment room, Jane's nurse, another lovely person named Deb, moved her to the bed. Because the drug had to be injected into her buttocks, we flipped Jane over. Mercifully, her face-down position would prevent her from seeing the obscenely long and menacing needle as it approached her backside.

Jane had lost so much muscle mass that I thought Deb might not be able to find a place in Jane's butt with enough bulk to handle the shot, but when I mentioned my concern—out of Jane's earshot—Deb assured me that it wouldn't be a problem. Actually, she'd have to find two injection sites because the only way to get the full dose of fulvestrant into a patient is through two jabs, one in each cheek. Poor Jane. The drug was dissolved in a thick, viscous liquid, and I watched Deb work up a sweat trying to push it from the syringe. Each injection seemed to last forever, but Jane channeled St. Sebastian and tolerated her agony surprisingly well. When she was done, we reversed our route and sneaked back out of the hospital.

Jane hadn't said anything to me about her expectations for this drug; she never talked much about any hopes she might have for Eric's treatments. I, however, had decidedly mixed feelings right from the start. As soon as it became clear that Jane would survive her pulmonary embolus, I found myself thinking about how futile that victory would be given the fact that her cancer would soon kill her. I cycled through periods of truly unacceptable thoughts about how merciful it might be if her death were hastened. Since Jane's cancer was incurable, the only real escape from her torture—and mine, to be honest—would be her death.

The worst of these episodes occurred when she started fulvestrant. Our lives had narrowed by then to an endless routine of heparin injections, dressing changes, and macaroni and cheese. It was the dead of winter, when the sun sets in Boston at four o'clock in the afternoon. The world had closed in on us—wherever I went, I felt like I was trapped in a dense fog.

When I brought Jane home from her first injection, my obscene thoughts were: *What if this treatment works? Won't it just prolong her misery for another year? Another two years? Can't we end this sooner?* I'm ashamed to admit that I was referring largely to my misery, not Jane's. What a deplorable husband I'd become. I shook my head in an attempt to derail that train of thought and forced myself to imagine, instead, how even a minimal response to the drug might make Jane feel better. Too late, though. I'd entertained the horrible idea and my guilt was overwhelming.

A few weeks later, after Jane had received another dose, I was at it again. Nothing had changed—the sun didn't even seem to be setting any later. Once more, I wished I could know how much longer all of this was going to last. One night, I waited until Jane was asleep and snuck into my home office, softly closing the door behind me. I opened my laptop and surfed the medical web, looking for reports of clinical trials that tested fulvestrant in patients with breast cancers like Jane's. I found a few and read them carefully. Most suggested that, if someone responded to the drug, the effect might continue for about six months. Being moderately sophisticated about this stuff, I knew that some patients would not respond at all and others would benefit for years. But at least I now had a sense of how long Jane might last.

I ruminated about what I'd just learned as I stepped into the tiny shower I'd been relegated to in the guest bathroom. Standing under the pathetically weak flow, I felt another surge of guilt. How could

I possibly be doing this—trying to figure out when Jane might die? This was not what loving husbands did. I promised myself over and over that I would make no more attempts to divine how much longer she would live. The longer the better. Period.

In the end, my self-flagellation was pointless. Although Jane's symptoms improved a little after her first fulvestrant dose in January, she became weaker and more breathless a month later. A CT scan in March confirmed that the cancer had progressed again. The treatment had stopped working.

I was surprised by how devastated I felt. Apparently, I hadn't been wishing for Jane's early death after all when I was researching fulvestrant's efficacy. Just the opposite: I'd been whistling past the graveyard, superstitiously flirting with the reality of her death in order to push it away. Well, it hadn't worked.

Jane was now faced with deciding, yet again, whether she wanted more therapy. Eric suggested that she try a drug called Doxil, a more traditional kind of chemotherapy but one that had been specially formulated to reduce side effects. A measure of Jane's desperation to feel better was her willingness to give it a try.

Unfortunately, Doxil also had to be administered by injection—intravenously this time—which meant more visits to Dana-Farber. I was never certain that Doxil had any effect on Jane's cancer, but it sure did give her horrible mouth sores. They were so painful that she had to take opioids and was unable to eat for days. So much for minimal side effects. After a month or so of misery, Jane decided to stop the drug.

What next?

Eric had another card up his capacious sleeve: an experimental drug that might be effective against Jane's type of breast cancer. In contrast to traditional chemotherapy, which acts like a nonspecific poison, this new drug was targeted against one of the unique genetic alterations that was causing her cancer in the first place. Its specificity made it a little less likely to interfere with normal functions, which meant that it would not cause the typical side effects of traditional chemotherapy like the mouth sores that she'd experienced on Doxil.

The problem was that the drug had not yet been approved by the FDA—it was still being tested in clinical trials. But I had a thought. Jane's co-chief resident at the Brigham thirty years ago was now the director of oncology drug development at the pharmaceutical giant Merck. I knew that Merck was working on a version of this drug.

With Eric's permission, I contacted Gary, who was devastated by the news of Jane's illness. When I asked him whether Merck could provide its experimental drug for her, he reminded me that different drug companies often find themselves working on the same type of drug at the same time. He said that Pfizer's drug was actually closer to FDA approval than Merck's and that he would be happy to contact their head of cancer drug development on Jane's behalf. As it happened, the person at Pfizer knew Jane (everybody knew Jane) and was eager to help. Eric applied to Pfizer for permission to give the drug to Jane outside of a clinical trial—so-called "compassionate use"—and the company, with FDA approval, promptly gave the okay.

There was a lot riding on this new drug. Senior executives at two major pharmaceutical companies had extended themselves to make it available. Eric had worked overtime to submit the request for its compassionate use. The FDA had granted it. And then there was Jane herself. So far, she had greeted all of Eric's treatment choices either with silence or with skepticism—by not expecting any of them to work, she wouldn't be disappointed when they didn't. But now, for the first time, she confessed to a guarded hope that this new drug might perform a miracle—however transient. Jane was getting weaker and more short of breath. She wanted to feel better.

Up to this point, Jane had projected a determined fatalism about her cancer, never shying away from the fact that her disease was getting worse, never expecting that any treatment would delay the inevitable. But something in her had shifted. In addition to investing hope in this new drug, she began to express explicit regrets about her impending death. What was her biggest regret? It was that she still had so much work to do—so many more research questions to ask, so many more faculty to recruit, so many more trainees to mentor. All left undone. Talking about those lost opportunities brought tears to her eyes.

The fact that Jane didn't include me in the list of things that death would rob her of brought tears to mine. Maybe this was a sentiment she found too painful to face. Or maybe our marriage really was less important to her. I chose to believe that Jane was finding it harder to talk about her feelings toward me than her feelings toward work and that she would come to terms with her vulnerability in stages. She could start now by admitting that she was sad about the way death was cutting short her professional career. I anticipated—hoped, really—that as the year wore on, she might also talk about sadness at leaving other parts of her life.

Meanwhile, Jane wasn't the only one whose hopes were buoyed by the Pfizer drug. We were all feeling optimistic. I remember the special trip I took to Dana-Farber to pick up the drug when it arrived. I can still see myself standing in one of the back stairways in the clinic—the same one I'd run down seven months earlier when Jane had collapsed—as Eric's nurse handed me the pill bottles with a big smile on her face. I had a big smile on mine too.

Jane took her first dose that night. At each subsequent dressing change, I performed my nonchalant but careful assessment of her tumor masses. After about six weeks, though, I had to admit—both to myself and to Jane—that the new drug wasn't working. The masses were growing and Jane wasn't feeling any better.

This was the end of the road. Jane took the news well, but I could see that she was profoundly disappointed. Disappointment soon faded into resignation. Jane decided that she didn't want to try any more experimental therapies and she had no interest in conventional chemotherapies which, in any case, were unlikely to work. She was done.

When Jane gave up any further hope for treating her cancer, the pace and tenor of things changed. Life slowed down and became sadder as we entered a protracted denouement that lasted until her death.

TWENTY

Spring came late to New England that year as it so often does. I'd wake up on March mornings and look out our windows for signs of rebirth—buds on trees, a robin—but see nothing encouraging. This would go on day after day. I'd begun to wonder if something catastrophic had happened to the earth's axis.

Not only does spring take its sweet time in this part of the country, it's also a sadistic tease. After an interminable Boston winter with its dark skies and freezing rain, the vernal equinox might bring one or two days of sunshine and sixty-degree weather. Hopes rise and moods lift only to be shattered the next day by a nor'easter with punishing winds and yet more freezing rain.

The biggest fake-outs occur during April, especially on the third Monday of the month. That's Patriot's Day, the local celebration of the Battles of Lexington and Concord. It's also the date of the Boston Marathon, and the true fickleness of Boston springs can be appreciated by a historical survey of the weather conditions under which the race has been run. Marathon Monday might be eighty-five degrees and cloudless one year, then thirty-five degrees and snowy the next.

I know firsthand about these weather extremes because I ran in them. I must stipulate that I am not an athlete—I never played sports in school and I still can't figure out how to dribble a basketball. But I have a terrifying family history of heart disease and, in the 1990s, I

162

decided that I'd try to reduce my cardiac risk by taking up running. I wasn't particularly fast but I was determined.

An opportunity to test my doggedness presented itself when Dana-Farber fielded a charity team to run in the Boston Marathon. Team members had to commit to raising a certain amount of money for cancer research at the Institute in exchange for a slot in the marathon. This was devilishly clever. The Boston Marathon is not an open race. In order to run—to get a "bib number"—competitors must have completed a marathon during the previous year under a specified time.

Although these times are age-adjusted, they're quite stringent. I couldn't have run a qualifying time if someone had put a gun to my head and chased me with a pack of wild dogs. The aim of qualification is to restrict the race to serious athletes by keeping out pikers like me. But, if I could raise enough money for Dana-Farber, I'd get a charity number without needing to qualify. The lure of this back door into the Boston Marathon was irresistible for slow runners with big dreams, and the Dana-Farber program was wildly successful. It became the biggest charity team in the marathon and has provided millions of dollars every year for the Farber's research programs.

In addition to giving me an opportunity to participate in an iconic Boston tradition, the marathon was personally appealing for another reason. I'd become a serious runner around the time that Jane's behavior started changing, as she began her emotional withdrawal. The situation was frustrating, of course, because I had no idea why it was happening and couldn't figure out a way to reverse it. Meanwhile—this was years before I'd taken on the CSO job—it seemed as though my professional life was a morass of uncertainties. Would I get my papers published, would I get my grants funded, would I ever be tenured? These decisions were in the hands of others, not me. I felt completely powerless wherever I turned.

Although I wasn't aware of it then, I can see now that I threw myself into marathon training as a way of gaining control over at least one small part of my life. The strict regimen—designated running days, detailed mileage goals, rigorous documentation—provided me with a highly structured plan that stretched over several months on its way toward a well-defined reward. The contrast with the rest of my life couldn't have been starker.

I ran the Boston Marathon ten times as a member of the Dana-Farber team. To be truthful, I trained for it fifteen times but suffered season-ending injuries in five; I am more fragile than I like to think. I was a mere plodder but I finished every race I started.

As time went on, I got to know my fellow repeat offenders—other members of the team who had completed an unconscionable number of marathons for Dana-Farber. Most of them had run more races and raised more money than I ever could. Some were cancer survivors themselves, and all had been touched by the disease in one way or another. They're among the kindest and most generous people I've ever known. Oh, and I got to meet Uta Pippig!

Jane was surprisingly supportive. She would try to figure out when I'd be running past a certain point along the marathon route and then corral some of her colleagues to join her there to cheer me on. I couldn't believe she had the stamina to do this—she had to walk a mile to get to her viewing stand. But I loved seeing her there. I'd pick her out of the crowd—her height made it easy—then run up to her and give her a big, sweaty kiss. I used to tell her that this showed how much I loved her; I was willing to lose several seconds off my race time just so I could give her a hug. You don't see Uta Pippig doing that.

I was deeply affected by Jane's interest in my marathon runs. The bathroom floor incident—Jane's cancer revelation—occurred about midway through my marathon streak. I became adept thereafter at denying the cancer's existence but, at rare moments, the thought would appear unbidden that a time might come when Jane wouldn't be around to see me running the marathon. The possibility that I might someday pass her usual spot without seeing her there, without stopping to kiss her, was devastating. So, I pushed it away.

Even though I had run my last marathon in 2010, I felt like I was still part of Dana-Farber's team. So, whenever Marathon Monday rolled around, I'd watch at least part of the race in person to show my support. I planned to do the same thing in this spring of 2013. After the morning dressing change, I made sure Jane would be okay on her own for a few hours—she was doing well enough that we had discharged the home health aide—and walked up to the Dana-Farber cheering section at Mile 25 on the marathon course.

I spent about an hour at the race, high-fiving Dana-Farber runners as they sped or limped by. I was about to leave—I didn't want Jane to be alone too long—when I saw two rather stout Boston police officers in full uniform running as fast as they could along the marathon course, their handcuffs bouncing off their backsides with each step. Maybe they were on their way to help a runner who'd collapsed a few yards up the street. That sort of thing happens often enough during a marathon, so I didn't think more of it. I also thought nothing of the muffled booms that seemed to be coming from downtown Boston. Just part of the day's celebrations, I presumed.

I started for home, following the marathon course along the sidelines for as long as I could. It was my most direct route and gave me a chance to keep an eye on the race. But at Kenmore Square, about a mile from the finish line, a crush of people penned me in, blocking my way. Some were yelling about a shooting near the finish line; others said it was a bomb, maybe two bombs. A river of humanity trying to flee the area nearly swept me into a subway station. I fought my way back to the street and pushed on.

After a twenty-minute walk along the south side of Commonwealth Avenue that would ordinarily take only five, I reached the section of the marathon route where it dips under Massachusetts Avenue. I had to get to the north side of Commonwealth Avenue, so I started across the Mass Ave bridge. As I did, I looked to my left and saw an incredible sight. A line of Boston police officers and Massachusetts state troopers had blocked the marathon course. Behind them was a sea of runners who had been stopped in their tracks with only a half mile left to go in their race.

Something very bad was happening. I tried calling Jane to let her know I was all right, but I couldn't get through. I learned later that cell-phone service had been suspended in the area around the bombings. Being unable to talk to her only made me more anxious to get home. I continued fighting my way through the crowds and eventually reached our apartment.

Jane was fine but she'd been worried sick. Our building is only a few blocks from the finish line, and she'd heard both explosions. They rattled our windows. Jane saw the chaos unfold on television and didn't know if I'd been close to the bombs. I lay down on the bed next to her and we watched the news together for the rest of the day, devastated by the death and injury that had been visited on innocent spectators of what should have been a joyous event.

Shelter-in-place orders locked down the residents of Boston and Cambridge for the next few days while the Tsarnaev brothers were on the loose. One practical consequence was that the visiting nurses couldn't come to our apartment. Without Flo or Olivia, I had to manage the dressing changes on my own. It was awkward and a little scary but doable. The first day, Jane was skeptical about my ability to handle things without help, so she watched my every move with a critical eye. After the second day, she decided that I knew what I was doing and relaxed a little. Flo and Olivia were annoyingly patronizing when they heard how I had managed without them.

TWENTY-ONE

Heparin injections and tumor dressings in the morning, mac and cheese at lunch and dinner. The monotony of our sad routines tricked us into complacency. We were so focused on quotidian details that we didn't devote much attention to the bigger picture.

But shortly after the marathon bombing, things began to worsen in ways we couldn't ignore. The mass on Jane's chest was now producing so much fluid that the dressings we applied in the morning were soaked through by evening. So, I started doing a second dressing change by myself right before bedtime so that Jane would be dry while she slept. Just knowing that she wouldn't have to worry about waking up in a wet johnnie made her less anxious and gave her a better night.

Much more unsettling was the fact that she was fading. Mentally, Jane was as quick as ever and still enjoyed a rollicking good time with her nurses every morning, but she was having a harder time staying awake as the day went on. And I could see that the academic politics that had consumed her just a few weeks ago no longer held her interest. Perhaps she was growing tired of the fight, but that would have been unlike her. She was just getting sicker.

Meanwhile, I had been making a half-hearted attempt to keep my own career on track. After finishing the morning dressing change—we were usually done by ten o'clock—I would go to Dana-Farber, work until five or so, and then come home. This had been practical when Jane was well enough to prepare her own lunches or sit at her desk in the afternoon. But, by late April, she was getting weaker, making it harder for me to juggle the two parts of my life.

One Friday afternoon, I found myself in a richly appointed conference room at a downtown law firm where I was representing Dana-Farber's interests in a patent licensing dispute. One of my responsibilities as CSO was overseeing the department that licensed our intellectual property, hence the meeting with the lawyers. We were about an hour into what was turning into a long session—the sleazeball CEO of the company we were suing had just started presenting his thousandth excuse for not paying us the licensing fees we were owed—when my cell phone rang. It was Jane. I excused myself and took the call.

On my way out of the conference room, I lightheartedly asked, "What's up?"

I heard her say in a panicked voice, "I can't breathe.... I can't breathe...."

Jane was terrified because she was alone; we hadn't found it necessary yet to rehire the home health aide. As I listened to her struggle for air, I tried to figure out what was going on. Was the cancer in her lungs suffocating her? Probably not. I knew from her CT scans that it was growing too slowly to affect her breathing so severely. Instead, she seemed to be experiencing something more acutely life-threatening—perhaps a new pulmonary embolus. If so, she would be at risk of collapsing again like she did back in September. This time, though, no one would be around to resuscitate her.

"Hon, you have to call 911. Hang up and dial 911 right now. I'll meet you at the hospital."

"No! No. Absolutely not."

"But you could be having another PE! Please, let's just get you somewhere where you can be evaluated and taken care of."

"No."

"Look, if you're afraid of being intubated again, you know there's a note in your medical record that says they can't do it. You've made it crystal clear that you don't want to be resuscitated. I'll call ahead to make sure everyone in the ER is aware. But, hon, there's nothing worse than this feeling of suffocating. The ER could help you."

"No...just come home...now...please."

I knew better than to continue arguing—trying to change her mind would be pointless. I could hear the terror in her voice, but I could also hear how adamant she was about refusing any interventions. It reminded me of the way she had behaved when she was bleeding on the bathroom floor. I felt just as impotent now as I had then.

I apologized to the lawyers and made a hasty exit. As I hurried to my car, I thought about the speed limits I'd be breaking to get home to Jane and whether the cops who stopped me would be sympathetic. I needn't have worried—it was Friday rush hour and traffic had slowed to a crawl. My anxiety mounted each time I was trapped behind a line of stalled cars, watching helplessly as what should have been my green light turned red.

After an interminable ride during which I diverted myself by pounding on the steering wheel and swearing at drivers who couldn't hear me, I made it home. I parked the car, ran into the lobby of our building, and pushed the button for the elevator, which took forever to arrive and another forever to get to our floor. Standing in the hallway in front of our door, I fumbled with the lock. Using both hands to steady my grip, I turned the key, flung open the door, and rushed inside fully expecting to see my dead wife sprawled on the bedroom floor.

Instead, Jane was sitting at her desk playing computer games, calmly chewing Nicorette.

"Hi, hon," I ventured cautiously as I slowed my pace. "So...um... how're you doing?"

"Okay, now. I'm not sure what that was all about but I'm better," she said.

"Your breathing's all right? You're not feeling faint? No pain?"

"Nope," she said, her attention focused on the computer screen. "A-OK."

I watched her for a minute. She was right—she seemed to be having no difficulty breathing—so I went into the kitchen and sat down at our breakfast table. I cradled my head in my hands.

Of course, I was relieved that Jane wasn't actively dying. But this bizarre behavior of hers—*do I really have to keep dealing with this shit?* The insouciance that greeted me when I came through the door made me furious. Only thirty minutes earlier, she had called in a panic—first, to tell me that she was dying and, second, to put me in an impossible position, yet again, by not letting me help her. And now that she was feeling better, she was pretending that nothing happened. Was she kidding me with this nonsense?

But, as angry as Jane had made me, I understood that her behavior was a reflection of her new, more fearful state. Between the failed cancer treatments, the surgeon's decision not to remove her breast mass, and the need for more frequent dressing changes, Jane could no longer avoid thinking about the progression of her cancer and, necessarily, her death. Sitting at home alone—without an aide or a nurse or anyone else to distract her—I could imagine how those thoughts had started intruding on her consciousness. She might have tried to derail them with TV or computer games, but her usual tricks weren't working today. The terrifying thoughts kept coming— doubling back on themselves, intensifying—until she found herself in the grip of a full-blown panic attack.

Just knowing that I was on my way home had been enough to break the ruminative spell, allowing Jane to calm herself. So, in addition to being angry, I also felt terrible sadness. *How she's been suffering.*

* * *

Like Jane, I had been trying not to think about her advancing disease. Denial was a practical and useful gift—for a few months, it gave me the psychological cover I needed to be able to put in normal work days at the Farber. But now, with signs of Jane's decline becoming too obvious to ignore, I had to change what I'd been doing. I wanted to get the most out of whatever time we had left.

So, instead of rushing off to work right after the dressing change, I got into the habit of staying home and watching television with her for the rest of the morning. Jane made all of the viewing choices—I have countless episodes of *Say Yes to the Dress*, *What Not to Wear*, and *Queer Eye* under my belt.

Although I thought, at first, that my forced march through exploitative reality TV was the price I was paying to spend time with Jane, I ended up being totally seduced. I'm embarrassed that it took me longer than it should have to figure out that these programs are about psychology, not clothes. When I set aside my snark, I got caught up in the subjects' stories of low self-esteem—often frank self-loathing—and would marvel at the way the hosts could tear them down and build them back up using wedding dresses or fashion accessories as tools. I remember nearly being brought to tears when a hapless, beaten-down, twenty-year-old loser who was trying on a decent shirt accidentally ripped a sleeve and said, "This is why my dad says I can't have nice things." A few words of encouragement from the pros plus a killer wardrobe was all it took to make the kid feel like a million bucks, at least for the duration of the show. Jane and I loved this stuff. It filled our mornings.

At noon, I'd pop a Stouffer's mac and cheese in the microwave and let it cook while I toasted a bagel for myself. By the time I'd finished spreading the cream cheese, Jane's food would be ready. I'd spoon it out of its black plastic container onto a small plate, pour a glass of Coke on ice (her second of the morning), insert a bendy straw, and take our lunches into the bedroom, where we'd watch more television. When we were finished eating—sometimes Jane could handle a whole serving, other times only half—I'd collect our dishes and wash them in the kitchen. I'd check on Jane one last time, give her a kiss, promise her that I'd be back in a few hours, and then go to work. I wasn't quite ready yet to abandon the other part of my life.

* * *

Jane continued to profess indifference toward her family. Her brother, Tom, would call every so often, as would her mother, and Jane would speak to them whenever they did, but she kept turning down their offers to visit. Her sister, Sarah, would also call, but Jane kept up her inexplicable habit of being more annoyed than pleased by her overtures.

One family development during this sad spring did grab Jane's attention. Her nephew Bill, Tom's older son, was getting married in September in Los Angeles, and Jane quietly nursed the idea of attending the wedding in person.

Jane loved all four of her nephews—perhaps more, or at least more demonstratively, than she did their parents. But Bill had been first on the scene and, "from the get-go," as Jane liked to say, she'd been enthralled. It would be inaccurate to think that she wanted to play some sort of quasi-parental role—she didn't know how to be a parent—but she was certainly invested in him. Whenever she'd see her brother's family, usually at Christmas, she would set aside time to catch up in great detail with all things Bill.

Now Bill was getting married. Jane would have been all over the wedding plans whatever they were, but her interest was further piqued by the fact that his fiancée wanted a traditional Hindu ceremony. Jane was eager for details, which she got from Tom and then gleefully shared with me—the groom was supposed to enter on an elephant, but given their scarcity in LA, Bill would instead be mounted on a horse. The entire wedding party, including Tom, would be outfitted in traditional attire; Bill would have to learn how to do a Bollywood-style dance with his groomsmen.

The elaborate wedding box Bill and his fiancée sent as an invitation enraptured Jane. She had never seen anything like it. Under its ornate cover were baroquely decorated invitations to the rehearsal dinner and ceremony. Hidden below the invitations were tiny compartments with candies and other sweets. (Jane took private pleasure in the fact that the candies had been inadvertently left out of Sarah's.) Jane loved the box so much that she gave it pride of place on the oak chest at the foot of her bed.

Jane and I talked about how strong she'd have to be to make the trip to LA. Given her downhill trajectory, I couldn't imagine that she'd ever be well enough to travel, but I let her entertain her unrealistic expectations without arguing. She was finally showing an interest in her family and I was not about to let mere reality derail this happy turn of events. Not yet anyway, even though I was sure that, at some level, she knew that she was getting sicker. Her impossible wish was giving me a glimpse of her desperate hopes for health and life, something that she ordinarily worked so hard to hide. Needless to say, Jane never made it to Bill's wedding.

* * *

Our old habits ticked along to the extent they could. Just as Friday had been our Date Night, Saturday had been Movie Night. Jane and I loved movies, even though we couldn't stand going to the theater. Between the bone-rattling volume of the soundtrack, the obnoxious people next to us yakking through the rare quiet stretches, and, of course, the sticky floor, we saw no reason to subject ourselves to the horrors of the multiplex. Instead, in the very old VHS days, I would rent something from the video store; in the merely old DVD days, I'd order something from Netflix. Jane would have enjoyed the streaming era but she didn't live long enough to see it.

Not surprisingly, Jane always left the movie choice to me. Not because she didn't care—she cared, all right, and could be devastatingly critical if I chose something she didn't like—but because it was a task, and tasks were my department.

Movie Night endured through most of Jane's last year, and so, one Saturday in spring, we settled in to watch a DVD. I had chosen *Melancholia,* Lars von Trier's weird tale of a newly discovered planet hurtling slowly but inexorably toward earth. This was a gamble. Jane didn't like so-called experimental movies, but we had both loved *Dancer in the Dark,* an earlier, deeply affecting film of von Trier's, so it seemed a chance worth taking.

To be overly reductive, *Melancholia* is about a family's response to their impending doom as the looming planet fills the sky. The most moving and pathetic moment in the film comes near the end when the young boy's mother helps him gather sticks to make a magic "cave" that will protect them from the planet. They sit under their flimsy teepee as they await certain death.

Although I knew that the movie was about clinical depression and the relentless way it can overtake someone's life—the planet's name is Melancholia, after all—the longer I watched, the more I saw the cataclysm as an allegory for Jane's cancer. Just like the characters in the film, we were doing everything we could to craft a normal existence in the face of Jane's death. All to no avail. Even Eric's treatments had been no more than flimsy sticks that provided no protection against the collision of Jane's cancer with earth.

When the movie was over, I was shaken. I prayed that Jane had not made the same connection I had. I turned to look at her. She was staring at me, her mouth slightly agape.

"How could you do this to me?" she said.

I tried to tell her how very sorry I was, but she wouldn't speak to me for the rest of the night.

TWENTY-TWO

Despite objective evidence that Jane's condition was worsening, the "Groundhog Day" feel of our routines fed my complacency, making me willfully blind on occasion. So, in early May, when Jane began to complain of low-grade fevers, I was dismissive. But after a while, even I couldn't wish away the angry red skin adjacent to Jane's tumor. When my fingers brushed against it during a dressing change, she let out a little yelp of pain.

We told Eric what was happening. He thought that the mass was infected and that the infection had extended into her normal skin. This had happened once or twice before, and he'd treated it successfully with an oral antibiotic. Naturally, he tried again. This time, though, Jane didn't improve, so he switched her to something more powerful. Unfortunately, a frequent side effect of stronger antibiotics is nausea and vomiting, and that's exactly what Jane experienced. Now, in addition to her fever, her tender skin, and her shortness of breath, she couldn't eat.

At this point, the only way to get the infection under control would be to subject Jane to an intensive two-week course of intravenous antibiotics. She'd need three different types, and because of their potential for overlapping toxicities, meticulous attention would have to be paid to their doses and schedule. Unfortunately, the only way to do this safely would be in the hospital—the last place Jane wanted to be. By now, though, she was feeling so sick that she was willing to go.

I packed bags for both of us—I planned to stay with her—and drove to the Brigham. Jane was assigned a room in the Center for Women and Newborns, which was a bit unexpected. She would require a lot of nursing care for her chest mass and her intravenous lines, and we weren't sure how much experience that OB-GYN unit had with patients who suffered from advanced cancer. But any concern Jane might have had about nursing was eclipsed by her delight at being assigned to a room at the end of a long, dimly lit hallway. It was very private—a good place to hide from prying colleagues while she was an inpatient.

As soon as Jane was settled in her bed, a technician came by to place an intravenous line. When he was done, a nurse administered the first of what would become, over the next fourteen days, a constant stream of antibiotics. By the time all of these preparations were finished, it was six o'clock—dinner time. Whatever else this clinical unit had going for it, the dining amenities were impressive. It was an example of the marketing ploys used by twenty-first-century hospitals to trick patients into thinking they were vacationing in a resort instead of fighting for their lives in a charnel house. Jane wasn't fooled, but she did order a milkshake and French fries.

After dinner, we watched TV for a few hours until she felt tired enough to sleep. That was usually our cue for the evening dressing change, but I was pretty sure that the nursing staff hadn't been warned about the scale of the operation. This put me in an awkward position. In the same way I hadn't wanted to act like an entitled but ignorant family member when Jane was in the ICU, I didn't want to overstep my bounds in the Center for Women and Newborns. But the fact was that they were unprepared for the task.

So, I asked to speak to Jane's nurse. I told her that Jane's breast mass needed twice daily dressing changes and that the procedure was a little like post-operative wound care—something the nurses would be familiar with—but more complicated. I tentatively asked if she would mind my explaining how the visiting nurses had been doing it. She couldn't have been nicer or more receptive. So, I began by giving her a list of all of the paraphernalia we'd need. When I came to the maxi pads, I told her not to worry—we had brought a two weeks' supply with us.

She recruited a second nurse to help gather everything else and then, following my instructions, arrayed it all at the foot of the bed just like we did at home. I asked if we could change the dressing together so that I could demonstrate the process and both nurses politely agreed, saying it would be a great idea. I knew they were patronizing me but that was a lot better than refusing.

I led them through the whole rigmarole while they took notes. Those nurses deserve a lot of credit for maintaining their sangfroid when I exposed the mass in all its ugly glory. We cleaned it up together, then rebuilt the dressing—they seemed to get a kick out of the Stayfree Maxi pad step. I repeated the tutorial for the next two nursing shifts, after which they passed on the know-how to any new nurses who covered Jane.

After a few days on three powerful antibiotics, Jane's fever abated and her skin was a little less red and tender. Unfortunately, her IV lines kept clogging—it happened almost daily—forcing the techs to insert new ones so that she could continue her treatment. Jane was turning into a human pincushion.

The need for frequent intravenous access was not going to go away. Even when her current round of antibiotics was complete, Jane's future comfort—for whatever time she had left—would require repeated administration of IV drugs and fluids. Trying to accomplish this by inserting a new line in her arm or hand every time she needed another intervention would be torture. Something had to be done.

On Eric's recommendation, Jane reluctantly agreed to undergo placement of a permanent intravenous line—a so-called central venous catheter. This would require a minor surgical procedure in which a narrow plastic tube would be tunneled under the skin of her upper left chest and inserted into one of the large veins that led to her heart. The other end of the tube, sealed by a silicone plug, would remain outside her chest. Whenever Jane needed intravenous medication, a needle could be inserted into the plug. Drugs injected into the catheter would flow through the large vein into her heart and from there to the rest of her body. The catheter could also be used to draw blood so that Jane wouldn't have to suffer any more needle sticks for blood tests.

Although the catheter would unquestionably improve her quality of life, Jane was not thrilled by the idea. Back when she was doing clinical work, the decision to place this kind of permanent intravenous line was usually made when cancer patients were failing and needed more intensive therapy. It used to be one of the last way stations on a cancer patient's journey. In Jane's mind, Eric's recommendation had moved her into that unhappy category, and she stubbornly ignored his argument that these catheters were now being used much earlier in a patient's treatment course so his recommendation carried no negative implications. She didn't explicitly express her feelings, but I watched her become more withdrawn once the surgery was scheduled.

After eight days of antibiotics, the surgeons thought that Jane's infection had been controlled well enough for them to insert the catheter safely. On the morning of her surgery, an orderly helped Jane into a wheelchair and I tagged along as he took her to the operating rooms in the basement. He parked us next to one of the dozens of beds in the recovery suite where a surgical nurse was waiting. She guided Jane into the bed, went through her pre-operative check, and then told us to relax. She said that someone would be along shortly to take Jane to the OR.

I held Jane's hand while we waited. She didn't say much. I don't think she was particularly afraid, but her silence betrayed trepidation. So, I trotted out the usual comforting things one says in these situations—it'll be done before you know it, this is a great surgical hospital, in two hours we'll be back in your room watching TV—and Jane took my comments for what they were worth. I kept up my monologue, though, and I'm pretty sure I made her laugh at least once. I can't remember what I said, but I do remember thinking that it was the most effective intervention I had made in days.

Eventually, they came to take Jane to the OR. The nurses said that when the surgery was finished, they'd bring her right back to the same place, so they let me stay there to wait for her. I spent a couple of hours watching conscious patients being wheeled out of the unit through its big double doors and unconscious ones being wheeled in. It had an efficient, industrial feel.

At last, Jane's was the bed that came through the doors, and the nurses, true to their word, returned her to the empty spot next to my chair. I stroked Jane's forehead until she woke up. When she did, she didn't seem much the worse for wear, physically or mentally. In fact, she was in a pretty good mood—partly from a sense of accomplishment now that the surgery was behind her and partly from the anxiety-reducing effects of her anesthesia.

But the mood didn't last. A few minutes later, when the drugs had worn off a bit more, Jane reached up to feel the bandaged area on her chest where the catheter had been placed. On her face was a look of horror mixed with rage.

"Is this where they inserted the line? Are you kidding? I can't believe this!"

"What's the problem?" I asked. I had no idea what she was talking about.

"I told them to put it by my shoulder. They put it way too close to my sternum." She was talking about her breastbone.

"What do you mean? Are you worried about it interfering with blood vessels or lymph nodes in the middle of your chest?"

"No, no, no!" she said. "What if I wear a dress or an open-collared shirt? People will be able to see it. It needed to be closer to my shoulder so that my clothes would hide it. How can I go back to work if this...this...*thing*...is visible?"

Given the way she'd been declining over the past few months, Jane's concern for how she might look at work sounded delusional. I was hoping that this might be a lingering effect of the anesthesia. But it wasn't. As soon as we got back to her room, she asked for a mirror so she could see exactly where the catheter had been placed. I found one and held it up for her. She took a quick look and became even angrier.

"This is utterly unacceptable," she said.

I tried to gauge how serious she was by asking if she wanted to go back to the OR to have it moved, thinking that such a ridiculous suggestion would bring her to her senses. I was shocked when she said that was exactly what she wanted.

I couldn't muster the strength to argue with her—to tell Jane that she was being irrational, that there was no possibility she would ever go back to work, and that the location of the catheter was the least of her problems. Instead, I did my usual accommodation dance. I said I'd talk to Eric and the surgeon about the possibility of repositioning the catheter.

Eric was understanding but thought that a return trip to the OR was nuts, which it was. The surgeon cocked an eyebrow when I described what Jane wanted. After taking a beat, he said that he supposed he'd be willing to redo the placement of the catheter if that's what "the patient" really wanted. I reported back to Jane that the team was willing to consider another operation. She seemed pleased.

The next day, the surgeon came by to do a routine post-operative check on Jane. In the course of his examination, he told her that he'd heard that she wanted him to move the exit point of her catheter closer to her shoulder. He said that all surgical procedures carry a risk of complications, even a simple operation like this one, but that if she felt strongly about it, he would be willing to take her back to the OR.

Jane slowly shook her head and said, "No, that won't be necessary."

Another door closed.

* * *

Jane stayed in the hospital for seven more days to complete her antibiotic course. I continued to camp out in her room, helping with the dressing changes and bringing her soup from Au Bon Pain after she'd cycled through the gourmet inpatient menu. Word got out that she was in the hospital but everyone knew she didn't want any visitors so, thankfully, no one came by.

That was fortunate. Jane's demand for privacy gave us uninterrupted time to begin the difficult conversation about her advancing disease. Just a few months earlier, Jane would have deftly avoided the topic by turning her attention to the television. Now, though, as evidence of her decline became undeniable, she was more willing to talk. Mostly, she seemed to be testing the idea of surrender—not giving up, exactly, but accepting the reality of her impending death. She was trying out an attitude that reflected a shift away from active interventions—experimental treatments, surgical removal of her mass—toward palliative measures that would make her comfortable.

What this really meant, of course, was that she was thinking about hospice. Both Jane and I had tremendous respect for the hospice concept. Jane, in particular, through her end-of-life research, understood the role that it could play in a realistic and comforting approach to terminal illness for a patient and her family. And I had seen firsthand the benefits it provided my mother when she was dying. Hospice may be one of the true triumphs of Western civilization.

But a smooth shift from active medical care to hospice depends on a patient's acceptance of the imminence of her demise. I had assumed that the recent spate of bad news—the failure of her experimental therapy, the surgeon's refusal to operate on her mass, the serious infection—had helped reconcile Jane to her death. It had certainly made it more real for me. But Jane's visceral response to the location of her central venous catheter seemed to reflect a tenacious unwillingness to let go.

Still, despite Jane's unrealistic thoughts about returning to work, something about this hospital admission had pushed her a little closer to acceptance. At least she was starting to acknowledge that hospice care might make her death easier. As usual, her attitude was coolly dispassionate—she didn't cry at all as she talked about facing death. Naturally, being me, I took my cue from her and didn't blubber either. But the whole interaction felt false. On the surface, we were talking calmly about the end of Jane's life while, underneath, we were keening and rending our clothes. God forbid that any of that sloppy emotion should see the light of day. Such are the habits refined by thirty years of marriage.

As it happened, though, we knew someone Jane could be more honest with: a colleague who ran the palliative care division at Dana-Farber. Susan was a psychiatrist and one of the most deeply empathetic people I have ever met. Because of Jane's research interest in end-of-life care, the two of them developed a professional relationship that had evolved into a friendship.

Jane's illness affected Susan deeply. After Jane came home from the hospital in September, Susan would call every so often just to check in. Later, they got into the habit of talking on Sunday afternoons. If I happened to be with Jane when Susan called, she would shoo me out of the bedroom, reminding me to close the door on my way out. Jane refused to speak to anyone else who might have had the temerity to reach out to her, but she always took Susan's calls.

One Sunday, I came back into the bedroom to find Jane in tears.

"God damn it," she said. "I hate these calls with Susan. She always makes me cry."

And yet, Jane kept talking to her. Those regular conversations provided Jane with a stealthy way to engage in a kind of informal psychotherapy without having to acknowledge it—she always maintained that therapy was utter bullshit. They also gave Susan a way to stay close to her friend, someone she dearly loved and admired.

But now, with active interventions for Jane's cancer at an end, Susan played an important role in helping her understand how hospice could be beneficial. Susan also had connections. She knew the medical director of the Boston hospice, and she offered to make calls to smooth the admission process. By the time Jane was ready to leave the hospital at the end of May, arrangements had been made for hospice to visit us at home.

After hearing door after door slam shut, one was finally opening.

* * *

Never underestimate the potential for tragedy to descend into farce.

We were now ready to go home—saddened but with a clearer understanding of our future. Although Jane had finished two weeks of antibiotics and was feeling better, she was still quite weak, and I was worried that I wouldn't be able to drive her home by myself. So, I asked Jane's nurse if she could order us a chair car—a van with a hydraulic platform for lifting wheelchair-bound patients into the back. It's what we had used to take Jane home from the hospital the first time.

The nurse looked at me like I had two heads.

"You know...a chair car," I said encouragingly, thinking that merely repeating the words would provide sufficient explanation.

Her expression didn't change.

"It's a car or a van that looks like an ambulance," I tried. "And we can put Jane in it and they can drive her home while I follow in my own car."

Comprehension dawned. The nurse nodded and said she'd take care of it.

The hospital discharge process seems interminable when you're ready to go. After waiting for what felt like hours, the nursing desk called to let us know that we were all set.

I helped Jane into a wheelchair and then stood by for transport to take us to the chair car, which, I assumed, was idling at the hospital entrance.

Just then, the door opened a crack and our nurse stuck her head in.

"The chair car is here," she said.

"Fantastic!" I said and positioned myself behind Jane's wheelchair, ready to roll her out of the room.

The nurse opened the door all the way and there, in the hallway, was an enormous toy car. It was made of wood and painted in gaudy circus colors. It was just big enough for a smallish person to fit in the seat behind the bright red steering wheel.

"What's this?" I asked as I tried to maneuver Jane's wheelchair around the thing.

"It's your chair car."

With the best of intentions, our nurse had gone all the way to Children's Hospital next door to find the fun-filled conveyance they use to take kids around the hospital for various tests.

In the most non-threatening and understanding tone I could muster, I said that this was not what I had in mind. I suggested that perhaps we could talk to the nurse's shift supervisor to straighten things out. She fetched the senior nurse and I explained the situation. After another hour, the real chair car took Jane home.

TWENTY-THREE

Jane left the hospital at the end of May. By September, she'd be dead.

Until now, Jane's death hadn't seemed real. Of course, I'd had intimations when she was bleeding on the bathroom floor, and those intimations hardened into certainties after her collapse four years later. But the snail's pace of her decline and the monotony of our daily routines had made the end feel remote.

That had changed while she'd been hospitalized. Those two weeks at the Brigham were filled with so many harbingers of her death that it now felt not only real but imminent. Jane's attitude had shifted too. Her decision not to redo the position of her catheter spoke volumes.

When I began writing about the final months of Jane's life, my plan had been to recall as many events as I could and place them in their proper temporal order. I prodded my memory by reading old emails and used their time stamps to create a proper chronology. I tried to be a historian.

But that's not what our last, sad summer was about. We didn't live that time as a series of events. Rather, everything we experienced seemed to contribute to our evolving feelings about Jane's death and each other. We compressed into a few months much of the emotional work that should have taken place over the course of years, beginning when Jane first discovered her cancer.

Feelings are harder to parse than facts—harder to dredge up, harder to reexperience, and harder to write about. They stubbornly refuse to take their place in a tidy narrative. But life, unlike history, is not "just one damned fact after another." The significance of that summer—both then and now—lies less in what happened than in what we felt.

* * *

Although Jane had started to come to terms with her death, she was disinclined to think about it if she didn't have to. Unfortunately, events conspired to force her into facing the unwelcome fact more often than she would have liked. Most of these episodes were objectively trivial, rooted in mundane or practical matters, but they could produce devastating emotional fallout.

At the top of the list were the departures of Flo and Olivia. After months of caring for Jane, those tough-as-nails nurses had fallen in love with her. I'm sure that their feelings confused them. They were becoming more and more attached to this maternal, empathic, and funny woman who, at the same time, was dying in front of their eyes. Having to tend to Jane's massive tumor at every visit deprived them of an opportunity to suppress or deny, even for a short time, their knowledge of her eventual outcome. Still, it didn't keep them from loving her.

In return, Flo and Olivia provided Jane with a reliable, stable mooring to which she could return every morning no matter what horrible things might be happening to her. They were permanent fixtures.

Until they weren't.

Flo left first, quitting her job at the agency in the spring to pursue other interests. Jane was saddened by her departure but, at least superficially, handled the loss well.

As for Olivia, she stayed on and grew even closer to Jane. But after a month she, too, decided to leave. I found out about Olivia's plans while I was running errands one afternoon. Jane called my cell phone and when I answered all I heard was sobbing. I thought something horrible had happened—the mass was bleeding or she was having new trouble breathing. I was right. Something horrible had happened, but not anything medical. Olivia had just told Jane she was quitting and Jane was utterly distraught.

"Everyone is leaving me," Jane cried into the phone.

I rushed home to find Jane in a fetal position and Olivia lying behind her, spooning her. Both of them were crying.

The losses didn't stop there. Back when Jane was toying with the idea of returning to work, her main worry was that her muscle wasting would make her look too skeletal—hence the episode with Flo and the butt pads. But that wasn't her only concern. She had been bedbound for weeks and thought that her immobility might have made her too weak to sit upright at her desk or meet with people face to face.

Flo came to the rescue again. This time, she thought that physical therapy might help Jane rebuild some strength. So, she put in an order for PT and a therapist began to make weekly visits. Kathryn became another young woman who instantly bonded with Jane. During their workouts—mainly Jane doing laps on her walker around our apartment with her oxygen tubes trailing behind her—she would ask Kathryn details about her personal life and soon learned all there was to know about her family, her fiancée, her wedding plans, and more.

Like all the twenty-somethings in Jane's orbit, Kathryn was utterly devoted to her. So much so that when she was given an opportunity to leave her current job for a better one, she didn't breathe a word. But after Jane came home from the hospital in May, Kathryn couldn't hide the truth any longer and told Jane she was quitting.

Jane was crushed—yet another person she depended on was abandoning her. First Flo, then Olivia, and now Kathryn. The losses felt like rehearsals for the biggest loss of all.

Although Jane rallied after Kathryn's departure, she was knocked down again a week later. Jane had assumed that she would be able to continue PT with a different therapist but, because she was now in hospice, her insurance carrier denied coverage. Physical therapy is for people who get better; hospice is for people who don't.

"It made me cry," Jane told me after reading the message from the insurer. "Not because I need PT but because I don't."

* * *

It was clear when Jane came home from the hospital that she couldn't be left alone anymore, so I rehired our home health aide. With Barbara watching over her, I figured it would be safe for me to go to work in the afternoons. I tried it for two days, but on the third, as I was gathering up our lunch dishes before leaving, Jane stopped me.

"Are you going to work now?" she asked.

"Yes, I thought I would," I replied.

"Are you sure you want to do that? I mean it's pretty clear that I'm not going to last much longer. I would've thought that by now you'd want to spend as much time with me as you can."

I was taken aback not so much by Jane's request, which was reasonable enough, but by the explicit reference to her impending death. She had never talked so directly about dying. That's how I knew she was serious.

She was right, of course. I had been seeking the comfort of habit and routine in the face of uncertainty and sadness. But now that we were entering a different phase—the last one—I needed to stay with her for whatever time she had left.

I let my colleagues know that I would not be coming to the hospital for the foreseeable future. I told them that I'd stay in touch by email and take scheduled calls, but I could not be depended upon to attend meetings or deal with emergencies. Everyone responded graciously and promised that they'd accommodate my needs. Much of their generosity was motivated by respect for Jane.

Now that I was committed to staying home, I assumed that most of our time together would be spent watching television. Surprisingly, Jane had a different idea. After lunch on the first day of our new routine, she turned off the TV—an unprecedented act—and asked me to read to her.

What a great idea. When Jane and I first started dating, our bedtime ritual included twenty minutes or so of my reading to her before lights-out. I remember beginning all those years ago with *The House of God*, a thinly disguised roman à clef about life as an intern at Beth Israel Hospital, where we had met. The book is patently ridiculous but we had fun trying to guess who the real-life models were for its broadly drawn characters. It was also a bit of prep work—mostly by negative example—for Jane's internship, which would start the next year. Then, searching through her shelves, I found an old, thoroughly beat-up copy of *The Catcher in the Rye* and read that to her next. The book hasn't aged well but it made us both remember how strongly our teenaged selves had identified with Holden.

Reading a book aloud to someone is an intimate act. It recalls the tenderness and warmth we felt as children when our parents read to us. But this private ritual for two creates another kind of bond. Reader and listener are synchronized as the story unfolds and can savor its twists and turns together, stopping whenever one or the other wants to offer an observation and then restarting. There is delight in such a deeply shared experience.

* * *

Reading to Jane did, in fact, evoke feelings I used to have while reading to my daughter when she was a little girl. So, during my sessions with Jane, my thoughts would regularly turn to Anna. She had been checking in every few weeks to see how we were faring and, on each call, she would be her unfailingly empathetic self, choosing just the right things to say to make me feel better.

It wasn't just that Anna was kind. She also had an innate feel for complex medical concepts and understood the way they can contribute to personal tragedy. This was something she had learned through hard experience in her own young family.

When my only daughter told me a few years earlier about the new guy she was serious about, I felt a mixture of happiness and foreboding. I'd met a few of the lunkheads she'd dated during and after college and was unimpressed—as is the right, if not the responsibility, of a father. Then she introduced me to Ted. He was different. An elementary school teacher thoroughly devoted to his work, he was smitten with Anna, and she with him. That was the very best thing a prospective father-in-law could hope for. A close second was the fact that Ted's great-grandfather had invented Crayola crayons.

After they were married, Anna and Ted bought a house in Boston and their proximity was a catalyst for strengthening our relationship. We were brought even closer by a problem with Anna's first pregnancy; a routine ultrasound at eighteen weeks showed that the fetus had a serious heart malformation. The condition would require a cardiac catheterization soon after birth, two major heart surgeries before age four, and the possibility of a heart transplant later in life.

I was devastated. I kept thinking about how unfair it was that Anna and Ted were being forced to deal with this life-and-death challenge in the midst of what should have been a glorious event.

Anna turned to me for emotional support, but I think she also saw her dad as a source of medical knowledge and advice, and I was happy I could help. But our conversations took a weightier turn. The ultrasound had been performed early enough for Anna to terminate her pregnancy, and I decided to address this possibility directly. I thought I could provide her with a safe space to explore her options with honesty and without fear of being judged.

We spent hours balancing Anna and Ted's unlimited capacity for providing love and support against the potentially diminished quality of the child's life caused by his abnormal heart and the surgeries he'd need. The calculation was particularly thorny because the severity of the disorder varies from child to child and there was no way to predict whether theirs would have an easy or difficult course.

Anna decided to keep the pregnancy and gave birth to a gorgeous boy, my grandson. She's been a wonderful mother, which is no surprise, but also a masterful caretaker. I've tagged along to her appointments with cardiologists and surgeons. I've sat and worried with her while her little boy underwent major operations. What's been amazing is not just Anna's love for her son but her ability to grasp the complex medical details of his heart condition. From the start, she displayed a kind of intuitive mastery of all the moving parts. Frankly, her understanding is better than mine. In the end, she and Ted raised a remarkable young man who, if you didn't know his history, you'd think was just another normal kid. Which he is.

I often ask myself how this mature, competent young mother could possibly have been the same little girl I used to read *Peter Rabbit* to.

* * *

What to read to Jane now, thirty years after I first read to her? We decided to start with *Sweet Tooth*, Ian McEwan's latest. We were both huge fans and had read all of his books, so this felt like a sure bet. Unfortunately, Jane was less than captivated. Her reaction was not based on the book's literary merits—rather, she was unsettled by the fact that one of the main characters has terminal cancer. My reading was supposed to take Jane out of herself, not remind her of her circumstances.

So, I made sure that our next book would be less triggering but still enjoyable: Chad Harbach's *The Art of Fielding*. Although a dicey choice because it's set in the world of college baseball—sports were anathema to Jane—it tells a great story and what Jane loved more than anything else was plot, plot, and more plot. Plus, she thought baseball players were sexy. She loved it.

On most days, Jane could listen to me read for about fifteen minutes before her eyelids started to flutter. I'd continue a little longer and then softly ask, "Hon, are you awake?" She'd reply, "Yes, keep going." I'd read a few more paragraphs and ask again. Eventually, she wouldn't respond; she was asleep. I'd quietly close the book and put it on her bedside table. Then I'd leave her to her afternoon nap, waking her when it was time for dinner.

TWENTY-FOUR

After a few weeks, Jane began to have trouble focusing on our books. She might forget important characters or ask me to explain yesterday's plot developments. Her wavering concentration was not caused by her advancing cancer. Rather, it was a side effect of the drugs she was taking to keep her comfortable.

The symptom that bothered Jane most was her shortness of breath—the slightest exertion could leave her gasping. Occasionally, like the time she called me in a panic, she would suffer paroxysms of air hunger that made her feel like she was drowning. Her CT scans showed why this was happening: the breast cancer that had spread to her lungs was growing.

Eric had tried to alleviate this problem by giving Jane more oxygen through her nasal tubes along with a kind of inhalation treatment that restores normal breathing in asthmatics, but neither intervention had been very effective. That wasn't surprising. The inhalation treatment, in particular, is designed to reverse acute attacks of asthma. Jane's problem was not reversible—her breathing would never get better. Instead, what she needed was a strategy for palliating the suffering caused by her irreversible cancer.

Opioids are the most effective drugs for relieving the suffocating panic that patients feel when they are short of breath. Of the myriad choices flooding the market in those days, the hospice doctors thought that the best option for Jane would be hydromorphone, known commercially as Dilaudid.

But the question was how to administer it. One of the blessings of Jane's new central venous catheter was that it could be used to give her drugs. The free end of the catheter could be attached to a small battery-operated pump that would provide a slow, continuous infusion of Dilaudid. This is exactly what hospice recommended. Jane refused.

Again, she was conflating her experience as a patient with her remote experience as a doctor. Twenty-five years earlier, she had ordered continuous infusion pumps filled with morphine for patients who were at the very end of their lives, and she now recoiled at the association. She also knew that one of oncology's worst kept secrets is that when terminal patients are close to dying, they can be nudged—gently and mercifully—toward their final exits by advancing the pump rate just a bit. Although Jane had been coming to terms with her own death and was more accepting than she had been at any other time, she was not ready for the pump. It felt too much like throwing in the towel.

Lucky for Jane, she had an alternative that most other patients don't: me. As a physician, I could give her injections of Dilaudid on demand. Hospice agreed that this would be acceptable, at least for now. So, they sent me a shipment of hundreds of cartridges prefilled with Dilaudid, which I added to the pile of medical supplies in the Jacuzzi. If Jane were having trouble breathing, I could grab a stainless-steel syringe holder, unscrew the plunger, insert a Dilaudid cartridge, and reassemble the holder. Then, with gloved hands, I could flush her central venous line with a little bit of saline to make sure it was working and inject about a half a cartridge worth of Dilaudid. I'd follow that with some heparin to prevent the line from being clogged by a blood clot.

That was the plan, and it generally worked. I was home full-time now, so all Jane had to do was turn to me if I was in the bedroom or let out a shout if I wasn't. At night, she could hit the button on the intercom, and I would be by her bedside in seconds with the works.

Jane's response to her hit of Dilaudid was something to see. Opioids had always made her feel good—really good. On the rare occasions when she was prescribed Percocet, for her one root canal for example, she would carefully ration the pills to make them last longer. Jane used to say that the best feeling in the world was falling asleep and Percocet made her feel like she was falling asleep over and over.

It takes a second or two for blood to travel from the heart to the brain, and that's about how long it took for Jane's eyes to roll back in her head after I injected her Dilaudid. The first time I saw her do that I panicked—I thought I had overdosed her. But then, as her respiratory rate slowed, she would smile and open her eyes. After a few more deep breaths, she'd look up at me and mouth the words, "Thank you."

The Dilaudid injections were miraculous, but the way I gave them—a single push or "bolus" through her catheter—meant that their effects didn't last very long. Jane's body still worked well enough for it to metabolize the drug quickly and remove it from her bloodstream. Early in the summer, that didn't matter—Jane only needed her injections a few times a day and once at night. But by late July, her breathing had deteriorated and she was asking for relief every three or four hours. I was assembling and disassembling injection cartridges so frequently I could do it in my sleep.

After a while, Jane realized that this was not sustainable, so she reluctantly agreed to be hooked up to the continuous infusion pump. I could see the sadness in her eyes as she surrendered to necessity. I was sad, too, but we both knew that it would provide more reliable relief than my one-off injections.

So, hospice ordered her a pump. But nothing about Jane's care was ever simple—figuring out how best to use the thing turned into another flail. The pump had two built-in functions. First, it infused a continuous, low dose of Dilaudid to keep Jane generally comfortable. Second, if she were to feel more short of breath than usual, she

195

could press a button that would direct the pump—instead of me—to push a high-dose bolus of Dilaudid into her catheter. The button was connected to the pump by a long wire so Jane could keep it near her hand at all times.

This should have worked. Unfortunately, even though the dose of continuous infusion Dilaudid was low, it was enough to make Jane sleepy. This somnolence angered her—she felt like it was robbing her of the ability to experience whatever time she had left.

But for reasons having nothing to do with the drug itself, hospice could not simply stop the continuous Dilaudid infusion. Central venous catheters are notorious for developing blood clots at their tips. When that happens, the tube becomes obstructed and it's back to the operating room for a replacement. That's why I injected heparin into the line every time I gave Jane a Dilaudid bolus—to prevent clotting. But there was no way Jane could inject heparin into the line every time she pressed the bolus button. Instead, the pump prevented clots from forming by maintaining its slow, continuous flow of Dilaudid—blood won't clot around the catheter tip if liquid is constantly moving through it. But this constant flow of Dilaudid was exactly what was making Jane nod off.

After some head-scratching, I proposed a Rube Goldberg solution: two pumps, both connected to her central line. One would be filled with a saline solution, not Dilaudid, and could provide a slow, continuous flow of liquid to keep the catheter from clotting. The other would be filled with Dilaudid that Jane could activate using the button to give herself a bolus. As soon as hospice understood how the setup would relieve Jane's symptoms, they got right on board. That's why I love them.

Now, the headboard of Jane's bed was draped with two continuous infusion pumps as well as her oxygen line. It was complicated but it worked.

Hospice had also provided us with vials of Ativan that I could use liberally if Jane's anxiety about her shortness of breath wasn't relieved by the Dilaudid. And they'd given us some atropine, which would reduce her oral secretions if they started to interfere with her breathing. With all of these interventions at the ready, plus hospice nurses just a phone call away, I felt like I had everything I needed to keep Jane comfortable.

That this was all happening during summer was sadly ironic. We loved our summers and, like overgrown children, we wanted them to last forever. But knowing that they couldn't, we'd anxiously mark the march toward the dreaded fall by the comings and goings of important dates on the calendar: my birthday in July, Jane's in August, Labor Day in September. But the first event in the series, the real start of summer, a date free of any apprehension, was the Fourth of July.

Although this year would be different—no holiday supper of hot dogs and corn on the cob, for example—I couldn't imagine letting the fireworks go by without helping Jane see them. So, as the big moment approached—we could hear the "1812 Overture" through our open windows—I got her ready. I attached an extra length of tubing to her nasal prongs so that her oxygen feed would stretch to our viewing post. I pre-medicated her with extra Dilaudid and topped it off with some Ativan to suppress her anxiety at being out of bed.

Then I helped Jane into her wheelchair, covered her with a blanket, and carefully maneuvered her to the room with the best view. I had cleared a space in front of the window and parked her there.

During the show, I spent more time watching Jane than the fireworks. As usual, each burst lit up her smiling face with a different color. She was holding my hand and gave it a squeeze whenever anything spectacular happened in the sky. She forgot herself for the duration.

When it was over, Jane was still smiling. But she pulled me toward her and whispered in my ear, "Take me back." Sitting up in the wheelchair for twenty minutes had exhausted her. I wheeled her into our bedroom, gently helped her into bed, and sat with her while she went to sleep.

TWENTY-FIVE

As Jane grew weaker, her stubborn side softened. For months she had refused visits from family members and all but three of her closest colleagues. Now, she decided, it was time to let others see her. Not surprisingly, her invitations extended only to a very select group.

The first outsiders she allowed in were Michael and Christopher. For a decade, they had been perplexed by Jane's refusal to visit them in Indianapolis, but they respected her privacy and pressed neither her nor me for an explanation. Then came the pulmonary embolus and the truth. When I did eventually call them with the news, they were horrified and kept asking if they could do anything for us or, better, if they could visit. Jane put them off like she did everyone else.

But as July slipped into August, Jane decided that she wanted to see them one last time. She was bedbound by then and, in her usual state of mind, would have fought against allowing anyone to see her in her weakened state. But things had changed—vulnerability was the price she was willing to pay in order to buy time with her friends. Michael and Christopher graciously accepted her invitation and planned a two-day visit.

They arrived the next week. Entering our apartment, they gave me tight hugs in succession and whispered how sorry they were. I thanked them for coming, letting them know how important their visit was to Jane and to me. I led them into the bedroom.

As soon as Jane saw her friends, she broke into a huge smile. Michael and Christopher leaned over and hugged her too. They were so happy to see each other that, at least for a moment, their joy displaced the sadness in that miserable room.

Not until Christopher gave Jane his gift did tears start to flow. Christopher had taken up photography—I guess he didn't need the three of us to badger him into a hobby. Jane had seen some of his work before and had told him how much she admired it. Now, just for her, he had prepared an album of finely detailed portraits of the flowers in his garden. The photos had been gloriously processed. As Jane studied the pictures—each one more beautiful than the last— she began crying softly. Me too. I couldn't help thinking that the evanescent beauty of those flowers could have been an allegory for her fading life.

The next day, Michael and Christopher said that they wanted to take a stroll through the Museum of Fine Arts, one of their favorite haunts when they lived in Boston. I would have loved to go with them but Barbara had the day off so I needed to stay with Jane. Walking through museums with Michael and Christopher had always been a treat. They were so knowledgeable about art that it was like being escorted by private docents.

A few years earlier, the three of us had gone to the MFA while Jane stayed home for some reason. Because Michael and Christopher liked to organize their museum walks chronologically, we started with ancient art and worked our way forward until we found ourselves in a gallery showcasing art of the European Renaissance. Suddenly, we were stopped in our tracks. There, in a full-length glass case, was Jane! At least it looked like Jane. We were staring at a wood carving of the Madonna and Child made in Germany in 1490. The Madonna's face was Jane's. We didn't recognize the Christ child. The three of us had walked through that gallery countless times and had never noticed the resemblance. It was an uncanny experience.

I had taken a picture of the carving, and now, when our friends returned from the museum to say their last goodbyes to Jane, I passed my phone around. Michael and Christopher laughed as they recalled our first encounter with "Jane as Madonna." Jane, of course, said that the carving looked nothing like her.

After a few more hugs and tears, they left for the airport. I sat in silence with Jane for the rest of the evening watching TV. Only later did I learn from Michael and Christopher that, when I was briefly out of the room, she had made them promise to look after me when she was gone.

* * *

I was caught off guard when Anna asked if she could say goodbye to Jane.

It wasn't her kindness that surprised me—Anna's empathy had only deepened in her adulthood—it was her capacity for forgiveness. She was moved to do something tender and kind despite Jane's decades of disinterest in engaging with her. Medical crises can bring families together—my grandson's heart problems had strengthened my bond with my daughter. Now, as Jane's death approached, Anna wanted to honor my love for my wife and temper my impending loss with a meaningful gesture. She wanted to be kind to Jane but she also knew that saying goodbye to her would be a gift for me.

When I asked Jane if Anna could visit, she said no.

* * *

In contrast, Jane decided that she was ready to take on the emotionally fraught task of dealing with her own family. This was a relief. I had been worried that she was going to die without giving them a chance to see her. She was now willing to grant them an audience but insisted that they not all come at once. Jane said that would have felt too much like a wake. So, they agreed to spread their visits over what was left of the summer.

Jane had the easiest time with her nephews. They were eager to see their aunt and, in anticipation, had sent her endearing emails recounting favorite memories. Several had to do with the way she would license their wild behavior during our Christmas visits to Michigan.

I'm sure the boys—now young men—were disconcerted by Jane's receiving them in bed, hooked up to oxygen tubing and infusion pumps. But that didn't keep them from enjoying themselves. I heard lots of laughter coming from the bedroom. Jane had mustered all of her strength so that she could be the brilliant, funny, and irreverent aunt they loved. Bill, Tom's older son, was accompanied by his fiancée—she of the Indian wedding box—and was proud to show Jane off to her.

Of course, being in bed and on Dilaudid while receiving Bill and his fiancée finally forced Jane to admit to herself that she couldn't go to their wedding. After they left, she told me to put the wedding box in another room where she couldn't see it. She didn't want to talk about it anymore.

In late August, Jane's brother, Tom, and his wife, Elizabeth, arranged their trip. I picked them up at the airport and brought them back to our place. Tom is a reserved man, and although I could see that he was shocked by the way Jane looked, he worked hard not to show it. Jane tried to give the impression that Tom's visit hadn't carried much emotional weight but, in fact, it was extraordinarily important to her.

Meanwhile, their ninety-four-year-old mother, Fran, had been begging Jane to let her come for nearly a year. Traveling to Boston would be a daunting physical challenge but she insisted that she needed to see her daughter and was willing to pay any price. Jane felt like she'd be paying a price too—more emotional than physical—but at some level, she wanted to see her mother and she knew that she had to.

First, though, Jane said that "we" had to make her bedroom presentable.

Fourteen years earlier, right after we moved into our new apartment, we hired a decorator who helped us choose furniture, rugs, and drapes for the common areas. The living room, dining room, kitchen, and main hallway soon started looking respectable enough. But then Jane ran out of steam; she halted the makeover before we could get to the bedroom. All these years later, we were still using the flimsy old armoire we'd bought on the cheap when she was an intern. Our bed was the same uncomfortable wrought-iron behemoth Jane had found discarded on the street when she was in college. Our bedside tables were rickety, unmatched pieces from Pier 1, and the side table was a round piece of wood balanced precariously on a stereo loudspeaker. That's where I ate my lunches while sitting on an ancient office chair, watching the flat-screen TV atop the armoire. The pièce de résistance was the carpet—an off-white number purchased in 1984, which had since acquired a complex patina of coffee stains and ground-in pieces of chewed Nicorette.

For years, Jane had rebuffed my entreaties to address the disaster that was our bedroom. It wasn't as if she thought that its current state was acceptable—she acknowledged that it was a dump. Rather, she thought that the disruption caused by a redo would make her miserable and that living undisturbed in squalor would make her marginally less miserable.

Now, though, the bedroom's decrepit state and the neglect it implied would be on display for her mother to see. It embarrassed Jane. So, with Fran's visit only two weeks away, Jane started issuing orders like Eisenhower invading Normandy. First, the carpet. Jane had me fetch my laptop, and I watched as she scrolled through every selection offered by Macy's, Bloomingdale's, and a half dozen other retailers. After hours of careful deliberation, she made a visually non-aggressive choice and had me pay extra for rush delivery.

While we waited for the carpet to arrive, Jane sent me to lighting stores. We needed a large shade to replace the torn one on the standing lamp next to the armoire, and two smaller shades for the lamps on the bedside tables. Jane still had to see every option before she could make a decision, so I emailed dozens of pictures for her consideration.

Finally, she wanted something nice on the walls—artwork or photographs. Dana-Farber was raising money at the time by offering framed artwork for sale, so I combed through the limited selection and bought three inoffensive prints that Jane found acceptable.

The new carpet was delivered with forty-eight hours to spare. There was no way I could switch it for the old one myself, so I offered to pay our building's superintendent to give me a hand. He was willing, but when he compared the size of the carpet to my minimal upper body musculature, he diplomatically suggested that he'd need more help, so he enlisted his friend, another super at a building up the street. They made a great team. I got Jane out of bed and wheeled her into the guest bedroom while they rolled up the old carpet and laid down the new one. The three of us then repositioned the wrought-iron monstrosity that was Jane's bed on the new carpet. After they left, I brought Jane back and helped her into it.

She knew that we hadn't done much more than put lipstick on a pig—the bedroom still looked horrible. But between the new carpet, the lampshades, and the wall hangings, there were enough improvements to satisfy her.

* * *

By focusing her attention on fixing up the bedroom, Jane could put off dealing with the emotional impact of her mother's visit. She clearly wanted to see Fran—the invitation had been Jane's idea—but how could she reconcile that wish with a lifetime of keeping her mother at arm's length? Worrying about carpets and lampshades was an efficient strategy for deferring introspection, at least for a while. Even so, the frequency of Jane's requests for intravenous Ativan increased as the reunion neared.

Emotions aside, Fran's visit also presented several logistical challenges. Not least was Fran's age, which made air travel arduous—she hadn't been on a plane in years. So, Jane's sister, Sarah, who was living in New York City, flew to Detroit, drove up to Ann Arbor to collect her mom, then drove her back to Detroit where they got on a flight to Boston. One of Sarah's sons, Gabe, came along to provide emotional protection for his mom and to see his dying aunt.

Given the complicated domestic and medical state of affairs in our apartment, as well as Jane's skittishness about being close to her family, I had arranged for Fran, Sarah, and Gabe to stay at a nearby hotel. I was not particularly happy about that. We would be making a near-centenarian travel a half-dozen city blocks to see her dying daughter. Granted, I'd be driving her back and forth, but it might have made more sense to put Fran up in our guest bedroom—now my bedroom—so that she'd only have to walk down the hall to see Jane. I could have easily camped out on the living room sofa for a few nights. But this was not what Jane wanted. It was hard to know who merited the greater accommodation, the dying daughter or her elderly mother. The coin toss went to Jane.

The flight to Boston was mercifully uneventful but it had been exhausting, so everyone went straight from the airport to their hotel for the night. I picked them up the next morning and we drove the short distance back to our building. As we rode up in the elevator, Sarah and I pledged our commitment to project bonhomie, so we were all smiles and eager anticipation as we entered the apartment. But then I ushered them into the bedroom. I couldn't imagine Fran's thoughts when she saw her daughter lying in bed, tubes leading from her gaunt face to the humming oxygen generator next to the bed, intravenous lines snaking from her chest to pumps hanging on the bedposts. This is the stuff of a mother's nightmares.

"Oh, Jane," Fran said, her voice breaking as she bent over to hug her.

They cried in each other's arms. After a minute or so, Fran slowly straightened up. I moved a chair next to the bed so she could sit down. Sarah leaned over Jane on the other side and gave her a hug. Sarah, too, was crying. She sat on the bed next to Jane. Gabe and I stood to one side.

I was included for part of the visit and got to see how a mother and her daughters used happy memories—with their mixture of laughter and pathos—to keep tragedy at bay. After a while, though, Sarah suggested that we leave Jane and her mother alone. She, Gabe, and I went on a long walk.

By the time we got back, Fran said that she was tired and needed to go back to the hotel. She and Sarah started the painful process of saying their final goodbyes. The scene was heart-wrenching. They were parting forever, with things that had long been left unsaid staying that way and unasked questions remaining unanswered. But Fran had done what she meant to do. She had held her daughter one last time and was on her way home to await what no parent thinks of waiting for: the death of her child.

TWENTY-SIX

Jane's last few weeks run together in memory. We were still doing two dressing changes every day but they had become more difficult. Jane was so drowsy from her Dilaudid that the nurse would have to hold her up in a sitting position while I wrapped or unwrapped the bandages. Jane, with her head lolling on her shoulder, seemed only dimly aware of what we were doing.

I never got to know the nurses who were with us toward the end. Flo and Olivia were long gone and Jane's somnolence prevented her from charming the new nurses. If Jane didn't bond with them, neither would I. I can't even remember their names.

By the end of August, Jane was eating less and less. She had lost her appetite, but she was also spending most of her time sleeping and had no interest in waking up to eat. The hospice nurses assured me that this was fine and reminded me that my job was to make sure that she was comfortable. I took my assignment seriously. With the help of the hospice doctor, I adjusted Jane's Dilaudid so that she wasn't short of breath. And whenever she'd wake up feeling anxious, I would give her enough Ativan to calm her down. These episodes occurred with decreasing frequency.

I spent almost all of my time at Jane's bedside. For a while, I continued to read to her even when she seemed completely snowed by her opioid. Eventually, when I was sure that she wasn't listening to me anymore, I would stop. But I'd keep the TV on and would watch it lying on the bed next to her. I remember very little of what I saw but

I do recall that *Men in Black 3* showed up one evening. I have no idea what it was about. Aliens or some such.

I spent my days and nights shuffling from room to room in a zombified haze. One thing I do remember is that three days before Jane died, a huge praying mantis attached itself to our kitchen window. That was weird—we were on the tenth floor in the middle of a city. Sure, there's a park along the Charles River behind our building, but a six-lane highway separates us. It's a mystery how that insect survived the flight to our window without being picked off by a hungry bird. Even more amazing, it remained rooted there.

I've always thought that praying mantises were incredibly cool. When I was a kid, my friends and I used to spend our summers in the fields around our subdivision hunting for frogs and exotic insects. A praying mantis was the prize of prizes.

Seeing that elegant beast where it clearly didn't belong brought me out of myself a little. I said hello to it whenever I passed the kitchen window.

On the day Jane died, I was scheduled to participate in a conference call. I had been trying to do a few work-related things from home partly to fulfill my responsibilities and partly to distract myself. But Jane was clearly fading, and I didn't feel much like taking the call. Still, a promise is a promise. So, when the time came for the meeting in the early afternoon, I kissed Jane on the forehead and, although she was asleep, told her I'd be back in a bit. I went to my home office and did business for about an hour.

When the call was over, I went back to the bedroom. Nothing had changed. I sat down in the chair next to the bed and looked at Jane. A minute passed before I realized that she might not be breathing. I really wasn't sure. I looked carefully at the blue-patterned johnnie over Jane's chest to see if it was moving. Maybe it wasn't.

But Jane looked exactly the same as she had an hour ago. I got up and put my hand near her mouth to try to feel her breathing. Nothing. I felt her wrist for a pulse. Nothing. I felt her neck for a pulse. Still nothing. How many more ways could I look for a sign that she was still alive? I had run out.

I sat down in the chair and stared at her. How could she have died during the one hour when I wasn't at her side? The whole point of this miserable year had been to provide comfort for Jane and just when she needed it most—the moment of her death—I had left her alone. And for what? For work? I was going to regret this for the rest of my life.

* * *

I sat a little while longer then roused myself and went into the living room to tell our home health aide that Jane had died. Barbara asked if she could see her. I nodded and she followed me into the bedroom. After looking at Jane for a minute, she turned to me and said how sorry she was. She walked back to her chair in the living room, gathered up her Tupperware, and left.

I sat down again and called hospice. The person who answered the phone was sorry, too, and told me to call the funeral home I had selected at random a few days earlier. I did, and the person who answered that phone also couldn't have been sorrier for me. She said that someone would come by to collect the remains in an hour or two. The remains.

I couldn't leave the bedroom. It was almost dinnertime but food was the last thing on my mind. Also, I didn't want to leave Jane alone. The last time I did that she died. I couldn't think of what else might happen to her if I left but I didn't want to take any chances.

So, I kept my seat while I thought about her. Every so often, I stood and put out a hand to feel her cheek or forehead. She was starting to turn cold. That felt pretty final.

I let my eyes drift upward from Jane's face and saw the Dilaudid pumps hanging by their straps from the bedpost. They were still on, so I turned them off and detached them from her central venous catheter. While I was at it, I removed the oxygen tubing from Jane's nose and turned off the generator. Then I sat down again and looked at her, now detached from her medical supports. She looked both better and worse.

Eventually, two people from the funeral home arrived. The older one offered his condolences while the younger one wheeled a gurney into the bedroom and parked it next to the bed. He gently suggested that I might want to wait outside while they prepared Jane for transport to the funeral home.

As I walked to the living room, I thought about the logistics of moving her. They'd have to put her into some kind of body bag and lift her onto the gurney. I mentally traced their route out of the bedroom and into the hall. I lingered on the tight curves they'd have to negotiate, the same ones that had challenged me when I brought Jane home a year ago. Then the elevator. There's no way the gurney could fit horizontally into the elevator. They'd have to tilt it on its end. Which meant they'd have to tilt Jane's body on end too. Grotesque.

The guys from the funeral home eventually emerged from the hallway, pushing the gurney with its concealed burden ahead of them. As I stared at the body bag, trying not to think about what was inside, the older fellow tapped my elbow. He held out his closed fist as if he wanted to give me something. I opened my palm under his hand and he dropped Jane's wedding ring into it.

I led the sad parade out of the apartment then turned and closed the front door behind me. I had no interest in watching them deal with the elevator.

I didn't know what to do with myself. I was dimly aware that I still had Jane's ring in my hand but stowing it was a low priority. Instead, I walked into the kitchen, which seemed like a good start to some kind of plan. As I looked out the window, trying to decide what to do next, I noticed that the praying mantis was no longer there. Had it left earlier in the day? I couldn't remember. I laughed, thinking it would have been a bit on the nose for it to have flown off the moment Jane died. But it was a lovely thought.

TWENTY-SEVEN

Jane died 360 days after her collapse at work. I had spent an entire year taking care of her. What would I do now?

The answer to that question would have to wait. I wasn't thinking about the future on the evening of her death—that was too complicated. Instead, what little focus I had was trained on the present. I sent emails to people who needed to know that Jane had died; I described myself as bereft. My cell phone rang a few times but I didn't answer it. I fried some eggs for dinner and went to bed early.

When I awoke after a restless night, I sought yet again the solace of routine by putting on my running gear and heading outside. I had two regular running routes in those days. Most often, I followed the paths along the Charles River—that was my favorite, but it's very flat. So, one day a week, I forced myself to run up Beacon Hill. Today was supposed to be a hill day.

As I jogged through the ornately gated entrance to Boston Common, I was surprised to see a lone bagpiper playing to no one but me at six o'clock in the morning. I ran to the top of Beacon Hill next to the statehouse, then turned and ran back down. The piper was still there playing a dirge-like tune I didn't recognize.

This is amazing, I thought.

The piper didn't know it, but he was providing a soundtrack for my mourning. As I passed him, I nodded in acknowledgment. When he started in with "America the Beautiful," I realized that Jane had died on September 10. Today was 9/11—that's why the bagpiper was there. I laughed out loud at my self-referential myopia and the piper shot me a dirty look.

When I got home, I stretched and showered. Over a meager breakfast—I didn't have much of an appetite, even after my run—I decided that I'd better start thinking about what to do next. It seemed to me that I couldn't plan for the future until I'd taken care of the present. That meant figuring out what to do with all of the things Jane had left behind, beginning with her clothes.

I couldn't imagine that anyone I knew would want Jane's used clothing so I decided to give it to Goodwill. I drove to a U-Haul store and, to be safe, bought more boxes than I thought I'd ever need. I brought them home, flat and unassembled, and stacked them in Jane's bedroom. I turned to face the closet doors.

When I opened them, my heart sank. I'd had no reason to look behind those doors since we'd started sleeping in separate bedrooms nearly fifteen years earlier and, consequently, no idea what had been going on in there. The sheer volume of stuff Jane had accumulated was mind-boggling. I felt like lying down and abandoning the project. But, I thought, the only way I could face this—and whatever else awaited me later—would be by harnessing the energy I'd been devoting to Jane's care while she was alive and redirecting it toward organizing her posthumous existence.

I began on the left side of the closet and worked my way methodically to the right. I would assemble a U-Haul box, seal the edges with tape, fill it with clothes or shoes, seal the top, and stack it in the entryway of our apartment. I was amazed to find that I recognized nearly every article of clothing, including jackets, sweaters, or shoes that I hadn't seen since Jane and I first started dating. I hadn't been aware of her hoarder tendencies but I was glad to discover them, in a way, because the old pieces evoked nice memories.

It took me three days to go through everything. I filled every one of the boxes I'd bought from U-Haul, including the extras, and had to go and buy more. When I was finished, they made five stacks, each taller than I was, and contained, among other things, forty-two jackets, forty-two blouses, thirty-four skirts, sixty sweaters, fifty-six scarves, and fifty-nine pairs of shoes. I know this because I had to make a list for Goodwill.

It was nearly a week before they could send anyone to collect the boxes. That gave me plenty of time to think about what I was doing. Whenever I walked by the stacks, I asked myself whether I should be giving away Jane's clothing at all. Wouldn't that be like losing her a second time? Goodwill would be wheeling what was left of her out of our apartment and onto the elevator, just like the funeral home had done with her body. I knew that didn't make sense. Still, the boxes of clothing were doing a good job standing in for Jane.

When the guys from Goodwill finally came, I didn't stand in their way.

Next up was the master bath, where the Jacuzzi was still filled to the brim with medical supplies. I began by stuffing unused heparin syringes into a biohazard container meant for discarding needles. Then, I gathered up the leftover vials of Dilaudid and Ativan and gave them to the hospice nurse when she came to collect the pumps. I filled a half-dozen garbage bags with gloves, bandages, gauze, and maxi pads. As I worked, the pile slowly sank—it looked like the tub's contents were going down the drain. Finally, I removed the hospital seat from the shower stall and restored the old shower head.

I was excited about using that shower again; I had grown thoroughly sick and tired of the tiny one in the guest bathroom. At first, stepping into that enormous shower stall was a glorious experience. But whenever I closed my eyes, I could see Jane, all skin and bones, sitting precisely where I was now standing, a trash bag keeping her surgical dressing dry. It was several weeks before I could take a shower without automatically thinking about her.

I had no such success with the master bedroom. Sleeping in the wrought-iron bed where Jane had died was far too horrible to contemplate, so I continued to use my old bed in the guest room. I did strip her bed and dispose of the bedclothes, but it seemed wrong to make it up again. Who would the fresh sheets and pillowcases be for?

But that meant leaving the naked mattress on the bed. It was covered with a smattering of blood and other stains—a grotesque visual record of Jane's final year—which made me not want to be anywhere near it. In fact, after I was done with the closets, I avoided the master bedroom altogether. It took a complete demolition job and renovation of the apartment—including the bedroom, finally— before I was comfortable in that room again.

* * *

Once I'd disposed of Jane's clothes, I was ready to deal with everything else: books, papers, pictures, tchotchkes. Even though I'd been dreading the emotional toll these personal items were going to take, part of me was looking forward to rooting through them. I was still struggling to understand why Jane had decided to hide her breast cancer. Maybe the papers she had stuffed haphazardly into her filing cabinets would yield clues, her hoarder tendencies working to my advantage.

It was a fool's errand. While a few items were interesting—especially those that shed light on Jane's history before we met—they told me absolutely nothing about her inner life. A perfect example was the handful of letters her father had written to her when she was in college. They were filled with quotidian details, nothing profound, and it wasn't obvious why she had kept these and not the dozens of others he must have sent.

It was the same with the few letters she had saved from Tom and Sarah. They were perfectly nice, even loving, but told me nothing about Jane. I bundled them up and returned them to her siblings. I noticed that there were no letters from her mother. Why, I wondered? Our keepsakes are curated—we make choices, consciously or not, about what to hold on to and what to discard. Perhaps Jane was more inclined to push away her mother than her father. Or maybe I'm overinterpreting things and Fran just wasn't a writer.

There were almost no letters from friends. This seemed consistent with the unsentimental Jane I knew. The only exceptions were two letters from Jamie Bernstein, Leonard's daughter, who had been Jane's roommate at Harvard. Jane told me that they had enjoyed a close relationship as undergraduates and that she had spent a few vacations with the family. But these letters came from a later time when Jamie's mother was dying of breast cancer. They were beautifully written and moving, so on one of my trips to New York later that fall, I met Jamie for lunch and returned them to her.

All that remained was the detritus of a lifetime in academics. Jane had kept her diplomas, her certificates from professional boards, her offprints of research papers. I even found some random blue books from final exams she took in college. It wasn't clear why she had kept them—the grades didn't seem particularly good. I put everything into the trash.

As I closed the last empty drawer, I felt terribly let down. No secrets revealed, no insights gained. But at least the cleanup was done. I went back to the bedroom for one last walk-through to make sure I hadn't missed anything.

I had.

Partially obscured behind a closet door was an oddly shaped cabinet that I had overlooked on my first pass. Its front panel had hinges on the bottom and a handle near the top. I tilted the whole thing toward me—it moved as a single unit—and looked inside. Lying in a corner, all by itself, was a plastic shopping bag cinched with string. I picked it up and carried it to the living room, where I emptied its contents on the floor.

Piled at my feet were loose papers, birthday greetings, and other ephemera. I knelt down and began sifting. Right away, I recognized dozens of items I had given Jane over the years—from little things I wrote when we first started dating to postcards I gave her last year.

I have a sentimental side. It's what makes me keep stuff like Jane's Valentine's Day arts and crafts projects and the kitschy airport gifts she'd bring home for me when she traveled. One of the reasons I had felt so let down after going through Jane's office was that I hadn't found anything she'd kept other than a few of my airport gifts to her. I'd shrugged it off, assuming that my memorabilia had been victims of the same lack of sentimentality that drove her to toss letters from friends.

I was wrong. She had kept it all—the clever things, the dumb things, the birthday cards, the notes scribbled for no reason. Every slip of paper had been important enough for Jane to hold on to. Their meaning seemed to inhere solely in the fact that they'd come from me.

But nothing with Jane was ever simple. Mixed in with my stuff were letters from old boyfriends. Jane had told me about those guys—I encountered no new characters as I went through the material—but I did feel a little threatened by the fact that she'd held on to their letters too. At least my cards and notes easily outnumbered theirs—I did have the advantage of being with Jane for thirty years.

I decided not to let the old boyfriends bother me. Novels from the pre-email era are filled with female characters whose old love letters are tied with a velvet ribbon and secreted behind a false front in their escritoires. This was no different—just not as classy. In the end, Jane spent half of her life with me, not them. I had won.

A little harder to handle was the last thing I found in the bag: an appointment book from 1978, the year Jane returned to Cambridge to take her pre-med classes. It had a black plastic cover and, on the pages inside, each day was allotted a two-by-two-inch blank square. Jane had used it as a diary. For the first six months of the year, she documented important events in neat, minuscule handwriting.

Many of those events were sexual encounters. After a perfunctory comment about her classes—a test in one course, a special seminar in another—she'd write about someone she'd met at school or at a party. The entry would end with a description of sex later in the evening. Some hookups were pleasant, others disappointing, but the brief narrative was impressively evocative given the space constraints. They were like sexual haikus.

On one hand, I could read these entries with a smile. It was the seventies. Jane was unattached and living by herself. Her diary was evidence of an independent young woman's embrace of her sexuality. Good for her.

On the other hand, she hadn't told me about any of this. Like all new lovers, we'd confessed our sexual histories to each other with a combination of shyness and pride. Jane had seemed forthcoming about the men she had slept with and led me to believe that her list was complete. It wasn't.

Maybe she was embarrassed by this part of her history. I could imagine that she might not have been particularly proud of this string of casual liaisons. But even if that were the case, she could have told me about them, adding that in hindsight she regretted her behavior. Or maybe she wasn't embarrassed and had no regrets. I'll never know. Either way, she hid it from me.

This made me think about Jane's later secrets. Perhaps the diary was evidence that her approach to shameful, hurtful, or scary things was simply not to talk about them. That way, she could pretend that they weren't real. But, if that were true, why hold on to the diary? Her best bet for avoiding something that made her uncomfortable would be to get rid of it.

Had Jane simply forgotten that the diary existed? I don't think so. The contents of the shopping bag included cards I had given her during the past year. That meant that she had been adding to her secret stash regularly throughout her illness. It seems unlikely that she would have forgotten what else was in there.

I've tried to put myself in her position. Faced with my own death, would I do whatever I could to make the lives of my survivors—especially my spouse—easier or at least less unpleasant after my death?

I'd like to think that I might force myself to consider what they'd find when they picked through my material estate and take steps to get rid of anything upsetting.

The only catch would be having enough time. But in Jane's case, she had a long runway. The slow advance of her cancer and her final year in bed would have given her plenty of time to think about what she'd be leaving behind. If she did have any of these thoughts, they didn't lead to action, and I'm left with only unsatisfying reasons for her demurral. If she decided that she couldn't be bothered to take inventory and dispose of unpleasant keepsakes, then her selfish indifference is merely painful. But if, instead, she was aware of what was in the bag and chose not to discard the diary, then I have to believe that she wanted me to find it.

Why? Again, I'll never know, but I don't think she wanted to hurt me. Certainly, Jane could be thoughtless but, in our thirty years together, she had never been intentionally cruel. Instead, I think this was one of her last attempts to gain some control over her life. Jane had been deprived of all agency during her final year. Not only was she helpless in the face of her advancing disease, but she had also lost control of the narrative that she had spent a decade crafting. She was being poked and jabbed and medicated and was keenly aware that people were whispering about her. That had to be torture for someone like Jane who abhorred appearing vulnerable.

So, I would not be surprised if she drew comfort from imagining that I'd stumble across more of her secrets after her death.

"See?" she might have said. "You don't know everything about me. I may have died helpless and weak as a kitten with most of my secrets exposed. But not all of them! I was wild, I had adventures, and you didn't even know about them. So, there, Mister Smarty-Pantsy."

* * *

A few years after Jane died, I found myself having dinner with two of her classmates from medical school. Naturally, the conversation turned to Jane. After obligatory expressions of sympathy for my loss and a few benign reminiscences, there was a lull. Then one of my dinner companions spoke up.

"You know," he said, affecting a pointedly casual tone, "I slept with her."

Shocked silence.

"Are you serious?" said the other diner.

"Yeah," he replied. "Early during our first year in medical school I asked her to dinner. We went to some Mexican dive in Harvard Square then walked to her apartment, which I think was up near Radcliffe somewhere."

"And..."

"And I stayed the night," he continued. "Nothing ever came of it. We didn't go out again."

"Did you know about this?" the other diner asked me.

I laughed. Not a nervous, uncomfortable laugh, but a full-throated "This is kind of hysterical" sort of laugh.

"Not at all," I said, turning to the first diner. "She never mentioned you."

"That's weird," he said. "Don't you think?"

No, it wasn't weird at all. Having read Jane's diary, I was not surprised that she had kept other, later liaisons from me. But I did wonder if my private hell was to be informed every few years about another man she'd slept with.

TWENTY-EIGHT

I was blindsided by my sobbing. Not just crying but deep, uncontrollable heaving that lasted for five or ten minutes at a time. I can't remember ever crying like that, not even as a child. I had no idea I was capable of such a display.

It made me think of something I had seen—or, rather, heard—twenty years earlier. My parents used to winter in Florida in one of those gated golfing communities that looked like the village Patrick McGoohan couldn't escape in *The Prisoner*. One morning on the golf course, my mother, who was a heavy smoker, suffered a massive heart attack. She was taken to the local emergency room where she promptly suffered a cardiac arrest. She was resuscitated but remained comatose, and it was unclear how much brain damage she might have sustained.

I took the next flight to Florida. My father picked me up at the airport and drove us straight to the hospital to see my mother. She was still unconscious and on a ventilator, but her blood pressure and heart rhythm had stabilized. We stayed at the hospital until early evening and then went home for the night.

My dad was a distant, taciturn man. He'd had a difficult childhood—his mother died when he was a toddler, his stepmother resented him, and his father was a salesman who was constantly on the road. My mother used to say that he never saw how real families were supposed to behave, so he hadn't learned how to be a father who could be warm and emotionally engaged. Maybe. But I wasn't surprised that he said next to nothing on the ride home from the hospital and only muttered a curt "goodnight" before going to sleep.

The next morning, as I made myself breakfast, I heard a noise I couldn't identify coming from my parents' bedroom. It was a repetitive groaning sound. *Oh, no*, I thought, *is he having a heart attack too?* Then I realized that he was sobbing. I had no idea that he cared so much for my mother—overt displays were not in his repertoire—and I certainly never imagined that he was capable of such intense emotion. Of course, by the time he walked into the kitchen, he had composed himself.

Now, I was surprising myself the same way. When I let loose with my first bone-rattling sobs, I thought the sound was coming from someone else. The loss of control was frightening. But when the spasms were over, I found that I felt a little better, so I began to lean into them.

I couldn't predict what would trigger me. When word got out that Jane had died, I started receiving condolence messages. First, there were the countless emails, then a flood of cards and letters. I was surprised by how meaningful they all were. Mostly, I'd just file them away, but every so often one would make Jane come alive for just a moment and the sobbing would start. Or I'd see a program on television that Jane and I used to watch together and I'd lose it again.

My sobbing episodes gradually became less frequent. The last one occurred on the Fourth of July, about ten months after Jane died. I was on my own that evening, as I had been on most evenings since her death. My friends occasionally asked me out to dinner and I'd gladly go and even enjoy their company, but I generally preferred to be alone. That night I made myself an All-American dinner in honor of the holiday and settled down in front of the windows to await the fireworks.

With the first explosion, I was wracked with sobs. I had to stand up and walk away from the show. I missed Jane. I missed sharing things like Fourth of July fireworks with her. I'd never be able to do that again. After a while, I calmed down and went to bed. I haven't sobbed like that since.

* * *

My last argument with Jane was about her memorial service. A few weeks before she died, she asked me if I'd given any thought to it. I told her that I had indeed been thinking about it and even had a tentative plan. Because Harvard had played such an important role in her life—and because she was a professor at the university—I thought it would make sense to have an event in Memorial Church, a stately chapel-cum-war-memorial that anchors one end of Harvard Yard. It seemed like a fitting venue and I thought the idea would please her. I couldn't have been more wrong.

"Don't you dare do that," said Jane, shaking her head.

"Why not? It's the perfect setting," I said.

"It's too big. It will be utterly humiliating to have the place only half full."

I pointed out that since, of the two of us, only I would be around to be humiliated, I was going to go ahead with my plan.

"Anyway," I added, "you're wrong about the turnout. People will be hanging from the rafters."

Jane stopped arguing, so I don't think she really objected.

If it weren't for Deb, Jane's colleague and former trainee, there wouldn't have been a service at all. She was much more plugged into the Harvard scene than I was and, as soon as I told her what I was hoping to do, she knew all the right levers to pull. She also insisted on hosting a gathering after the service in her family's rambling Cambridge home, a five-minute walk from the church. I was worried that she'd be overwhelmed by the crush of people who'd want to show up, but Deb insisted that she could accommodate everyone.

Deb's attention to logistical details gave me the freedom to devote myself to planning the service itself. First, I gave a lot of thought to who should speak. I wanted to hear from people who had been important to Jane at different times in her professional life—those who had trained her, those whom she had trained, her friends, and her coworkers. It was no surprise that every person I asked to speak said that it would be an honor. I also invited her nephews and trainees to be ushers.

As much effort as I put into the speaker list, I put even more into choosing the music. It was a way for me to work on the service without having to think too much about its subject. After some internal deliberation, I assembled a chamber music playlist that I thought would fit the occasion. Deb put me in touch with a cellist she knew who was active in the Boston music scene. The cellist liked my choices—at least she didn't object to them—and recruited the other instrumentalists we'd need. In honor of Jane, there wasn't a pianist in the bunch.

As I had predicted, the service attracted a standing-room-only crowd. So many people from Dana-Farber wanted to attend that the Institute had to charter a bus to take them to and from Harvard Yard.

The service was magnificent and sad. Anna, pregnant with her second child, saw that I needed her support and cleaved to my side for the duration. All of the eulogies were eloquent, and everyone spoke with an affecting combination of sadness and humor. The music was exactly as poignant as I'd wanted it to be. When it was all over, Anna stood with me to receive an endless line of mourners who offered words of comfort.

After the last tearful hug, we walked together to Deb's house. On the way, I replayed the service in my head and, for the umpteenth time, reassured myself that it had been okay for me not to be one of the eulogists. I had decided against speaking partly because I didn't think I'd be able to maintain my composure and partly because the depth of a husband's loss is pretty much a given. People knew that I was devastated. I wanted mourners to hear how others felt.

But Deb's gathering had the wistful, lubricated feel of a wake. After everyone had helped themselves to food and a drink, those of us who lingered gathered in the living room. That's when I decided to speak. I stood and began telling stories about Jane. I talked about all the ways I missed her and how much I had loved her. I finished by thanking everyone who had attended the service for helping me at long last win an argument with Jane, albeit posthumously. A parade of friends and family, including Tom and Sarah, followed with their own memories.

The day's events had been a celebration of Jane's shining attributes. That was fitting and proper—a memorial service is not a place for nuanced portraits. But the truth was that Jane was far more complex than the person described by the eulogists. Only I knew the magnitude of the disconnect, and that knowledge had unsettled me all day. To be sure, Eric was privy to some of the details and Jane's smarter friends had probably made a few correct guesses, but I alone knew the whole story.

Not anymore. I've laid out the facts for all to see, including revelations that cast Jane in an unfavorable light. In so doing, I've exposed the secrets of a very private person, someone who prized loyalty above other virtues. In fact, spousal infidelity—in word or deed—earned her most lacerating condemnation. Even lesser acts of treachery merited near-biblical denunciation. Jane subscribed to a complex taxonomy of disloyalty.

Where would my transgression fit? Somewhere near the top, I'm afraid.

But this business of disloyalty cuts both ways: Jane betrayed me with her secrecy. It's taken me nearly ten years since her death to finally acknowledge that and to allow myself to be angry at her. It's also taken me that long to understand that I can also miss her and love her memory.

To get to this point, I had to think deeply about our marriage. What I found was that our story is important enough, moving enough, and human enough to be shared with others. Her family, friends, and devoted supporters may think that they'll never forgive me. But they will change their minds.

EPILOGUES

I.

After Jane died, I had absolutely no interest in "meeting" anyone. I didn't see the point. I figured I'd been extraordinarily fortunate to have one pretty good marriage—at least that's what I told myself—and I'd be pushing my luck to expect another one. So, why bother dating?

Some well-intentioned but misguided friends waited for what they thought was a respectable period after Jane's death before telling me about age-appropriate women who they thought might interest me. These were lovely gestures, but I politely and firmly declined them all.

I knew a few widows who also waited a bit before contacting me. They, too, meant well, but I couldn't imagine anything sadder than two grieving people joining forces. I didn't pursue these opportunities either.

So, I busied myself with work. I accepted every invitation to travel to a meeting or give a talk at a university no matter how distant. I went to Japan to drum up biotechnology business for the Commonwealth of Massachusetts despite suffering from just about the worst cold I'd ever had. By the time we landed in Tokyo, I was deaf in both ears. Because our group was on official business, we were scheduled to meet the ambassador, Caroline Kennedy, and I couldn't pass up an opportunity to meet her no matter how lousy I felt. Jane would have loved the stories from that trip. Of course, I had no one to share them with.

Life went on. I renovated the apartment. My crying jags became less frequent. My solitary existence seemed to be going pretty well.

Then, nearly a year after Jane's death, I received an unexpected email.

On the same day in 1983 when I met Jane in the ICU as she began her rotation as a medical student on the other team, I met her classmate Lynn, who had been assigned to mine. Lynn was a fantastic student, certainly the best I'd ever worked with. She was smart, funny, enthusiastic, and, although not relevant to her performance, stunningly beautiful. For a month, we worked together every third night. I supervised her as she evaluated newly admitted patients and I helped her prepare her presentations for rounds the next morning. I loved teaching her and hanging out with her in the wee hours.

Lynn's last night on call at the end of her rotation was unusually busy. We had admitted several sick people to the hospital and, in addition to working up her own patient, Lynn had made herself useful by following me around and lending a hand whenever she could. At about four o'clock in the morning, we were sitting at a table in the nursing station writing notes in our patients' charts.

"Can I talk to you about something?" Lynn asked, looking up from her work.

"Of course," I replied.

"Um. Not here," she said, eyeing the nurses. "Can we go somewhere else?"

The ward we were on was a long, straight hallway with the nursing station at one end and a window at the other. I suggested that we walk to the end of the hall. The overhead lights were off, so the only illumination guiding our way came from the flashing red lights on heart monitors that had been placed just outside of patients' rooms. The hallway looked like a landing strip.

We reached the window and sat side by side on the sill. It was dark outside and dark inside.

Lynn turned to me and said, "I have a confession to make."

I looked at her, barely able to make out her face. I couldn't imagine what was coming next.

"I've felt a strong connection with you over the past month," she said, "and I can't help wondering if we should do something about it."

I was stunned. Nothing like this had ever happened to me before. A smart, infinitely desirable woman confessing her attraction? To me? Really? I lost my bearings for a moment—I felt like I was floating in space.

Then I came crashing to earth. Serious obstacles stood in the way of acting on our mutual attraction. First, I had already started dating Jane. It was still early in the relationship, but I felt that I had made a commitment. Second, and far more important, Lynn was engaged to one of her classmates and the wedding was to take place in just a few months. I could not imagine being a party to the disruption of those plans based on our brief encounter.

I told Lynn that I was more than flattered by what she had said—I was absolutely floored.

"But," I said, "there are problems."

I started by telling her about Jane; Lynn hadn't known. Then I gently brought up her fiancée and said that it wouldn't be right for me to get in the way of her wedding plans.

Lynn took my rejection well—another testament to her character. We remained friendly for the rest of her time at the hospital and, remarkably, didn't feel too awkward about what had happened.

And that was that. Jane and I went on to have a thirty-year partnership to which we were both devoted. But Lynn's late-night confession had left a huge impression, and I found myself revisiting her memory every so often over the decades. In fact, soon after Jane's death, when I finally decided it was safe to see a therapist, the Lynn episode still loomed so large that I mentioned it to my shrink.

The unexpected email that arrived in my inbox eleven months after Jane's death was from Lynn. I double-checked the sender's name to make sure it was the same Lynn. It was. The subject line was "Living under a rock" and the body of the email described her surprise at hearing that Jane had died nearly a year earlier. Lynn's note was kind and sympathetic. She wrote about her memories of being my student with a warmth that felt familiar. I responded by thanking her for her lovely email and suggesting that if she were ever in Boston, we could get together and reminisce about Jane. Lynn was living in New Jersey then, right over the George Washington Bridge, and she made the same offer to me if I ever found myself in New York.

That's where I left things until a few weeks later. One of my responsibilities at Dana-Farber was overseeing a program that took care of the postgraduate fellows who worked in our laboratories and research centers—the "postdocs." To celebrate the program's tenth anniversary, we planned to give an award to a highly accomplished alumna. My choice, which was eagerly accepted by others, was Helen, a preeminent cancer biologist who had worked in the lab next to mine when we were postdocs. We'd been good friends but, sadly, had only sporadic contact since then. So I was pleased that, as a condition of the award, Helen would have to come to Dana-Farber to give a lecture. It would give us a chance to catch up and renew our friendship.

Helen flew to Boston the day before her talk. She arrived in the late afternoon, so I went to her hotel to pick her up for a dinner I had arranged with a few other people she knew at Dana-Farber.

We had barely said hello when Helen excitedly said, "Do you know who my best friend in the world is?"

"No," I said, having no idea what she was talking about.

"Lynn!"

In this outlandishly small-world story, it so happened that Helen's and Lynn's families lived near each other in St. Louis. The adults all worked at Washington University School of Medicine, and their children all went to the same schools. The families celebrated holidays together, vacationed together, and the kids had grown up together.

"So, Lynn tells me she got in touch with you when she heard that Jane had died," Helen continued.

"She did," I said.

"Lynn also said that she invited you to have coffee or lunch or dinner with her when you're in New York."

"She did," I said.

"Well? When are you going?"

I laughed and told Helen that I had very fond memories of Lynn but that, as far as I knew, she was still married and it would be unseemly for me to meet her. It was pretty much the same answer I had given Lynn in the darkened hallway thirty years earlier.

"Well," said Helen, "it may not be my place to say anything, but Lynn's marriage is a little rocky right now. I don't think it would be inappropriate for you to see her."

I said that the status of her marriage didn't matter. Lynn was married, and I was not going to get in the middle of that.

Of course, Helen was no fool; she had struck a spark. As soon as I got home, I emailed Lynn to let her know that I would be in New York the next week and asked if she'd like to have lunch. She agreed.

I tried to make things as easy for her as I could. I was staying on the East Side, but I made lunch reservations at a bistro on the Upper West Side since Lynn would be coming over the bridge from New Jersey.

On a brilliantly sunny morning in late September, I flew to LaGuardia and took a taxi to Manhattan. As the cab pulled up in front of the restaurant, I saw Lynn sitting at a table outside. She was instantly recognizable. In fact, she had hardly changed since I'd last seen her. She stood as I got out of the cab. We said hello, looked at each other for a moment with broad smiles on our faces, and went inside for lunch.

We talked without taking a breath for the next two hours. Lynn told me about the trouble in her marriage—she was now living on her own and likely to seek a divorce. I told her about caring for Jane and found myself describing details that I hadn't mentioned to anyone. Sharing these revelations felt like the most natural thing in the world.

After lunch, we hugged and parted. But something had happened. My excuse for coming to New York to meet Lynn was that I was going to the opera; my cousin invited me every year to the Met's gala opening. Jane had been thoroughly uninterested, so I used to take my daughter. Anna couldn't go that year, so I'd asked my sister, who didn't seem to mind standing in. As we walked together to Lincoln Center, she asked me how lunch had gone. She knew that I had met an old friend but I hadn't told her any of the backstory. After giving her what I thought was a dispassionate description of my afternoon with Lynn, she looked at me out of the corner of her eye.

"It sounds like this was something special," she said.

And indeed it was. Over the next nine months, I made several trips to Englewood, where Lynn was living, and she made several to Boston. By June, Lynn had moved in with me and, nine months later, we were married.

My life has changed in ways I could never have imagined. I'm in a loving marriage with someone to whom I am deeply connected. I've gained three stepsons, four new grandchildren—adding to my two whom I adore—and two dogs. My daughter, her husband, and her kids are crazy about Lynn.

This has all been utterly unexpected and not something I sought. But I'm reveling in it.

II.

Three days after Jane died, I went to the funeral home to pick up her ashes. I had no idea what to do with them. My parents had wanted to be buried, so there were no questions about their remains. But now I did have questions. *What do I do with Jane's?*

The usual answers just didn't fit. Scattering them over a beautiful vista that held deep meaning for Jane was not an option—there was no such place. She didn't particularly like her family's summer home on Beaver Island in Lake Michigan; she never talked about a majestic scene that had captured her fancy; she never even walked along the Esplanade next to the Charles River just a few yards from our home. There would be no windswept promontory for Jane's ashes. I couldn't invent meaning where there wasn't any.

What else might I do? Ironically, the only personal experience I'd had with cremation was Jane's father's. The family kept his ashes on a shelf in his home office. That seemed like a perfectly reasonable decision. It was pleasingly unceremonious—a sort of practical approach to the everyday realities of death. So, that's what I did. I kept the box containing Jane's ashes in a small bag on a shelf in the closet of her bedroom—the room in which she had spent most of her time when she was alive.

Although my decision didn't have any deep meaning, it was convenient. And it kept me from having to think any more about the subject.

Then, one day, early in my relationship with Lynn, she asked me what was in the bag in the closet.

"Oh, those are Jane's ashes," I said.

"You're kidding me," she said with a look of horror. "What do you plan to do with them?"

"Nothing," I said. "I thought I'd leave them in the closet."

"Well, I can't sleep in the same room with your dead wife's ashes," she said. "You really ought to give some more thought to this."

She was right, of course. It's not as though I had made a thorough list of the options for disposing of Jane's remains and then carefully determined that my best choice was keeping them in a shopping bag on a closet shelf above my shirts. After the conversation with Lynn, I did move them to a drawer in my office, but that was only a stopgap.

Goaded at last into thinking more deeply about what had been most meaningful to Jane, I found myself returning again and again to Dana-Farber. That was where she had spent half of her life, where she had fashioned a surrogate family of trainees and junior faculty, and where she had bequeathed a sizeable chunk of her estate to support those young physicians.

But I was stumped. How could I translate her devotion to the Institute into action? Then I remembered that the most fun we'd ever had together at Dana-Farber was serving on the committee that chose the architect for the new clinical building. It was a real treat to hear creative presentations from some of the most preeminent architectural firms in the country. Instead of our usual diet of chemotherapy and cancer cells, we could spend a few hours each week thinking about the aesthetics of buildings and the spaces they enclose.

Both Jane and I were mesmerized by one architect in particular. He sported the perfectly round eyeglasses that every serious architect since Le Corbusier has worn. He was spacey enough to make you think he was an artist at heart but not so spacey that he wouldn't get the job done. A majority of the committee agreed and awarded the contract to his small firm.

The committee then shifted its focus to overseeing and evaluating their concepts. Jane would become notorious for declaring that one of the late designs was "too pointy." She was outvoted, and that model became the basis for the new building. She eventually learned to love it.

Like so many contemporary structures, this one had an environmentally friendly roof garden that provided natural cooling and reduced energy consumption. The building's top floor was stepped back several yards so there were actually two gardens: one on the roof over the top floor and one over the lower roof, which had been created by the step-back. That was the answer. I would scatter Jane's ashes over the lower roof garden.

I was happy with my plan but knew that it would be a delicate undertaking. I had to figure out how to get onto the roof without drawing attention to what I was doing; Jane would have wanted this to be a private gesture. Fortunately, I had worked for years with the head of facilities—someone who had known Jane well. I asked her if she could give me access to the roof garden to spread Jane's ashes and not tell anyone about it. She readily agreed.

So, two years after Jane's death, on another bright and sunny fall day, I carried the bag with Jane's ashes to the penultimate floor of the new clinical building. My partner in crime was there to meet me with her master key. She opened the door to the roof garden and waved me through. She then stepped back and closed the door to give me privacy.

I looked out over the city for a minute, thinking about Jane. I took the box out of the bag, opened it, lifted the clear plastic bag with her ashes, and undid the tie. Carefully judging wind direction, I opened the bag and gently scattered Jane over the garden. I lifted my eyes again to the city. After another minute, I walked to the door and knocked on the glass to get my colleague's attention. She opened the door, I thanked her profusely, and we rode down in the elevator together without a word.

When something happens at work or in the news or at home that Jane would have cared about, I return to the floor in the new building where the windows look out over the roof garden. I stand there, next to Jane's final resting place, and think about what she would have said.

ACKNOWLEDGMENTS

First and foremost, I must thank Lynn White for insisting that I write this memoir and for her forbearance while I was immersed in memories of my life with Jane. I am also grateful to Sarah and Tom Weeks for allowing me to tell difficult stories about the sister they loved. And, of course, I thank Anna Wells for never losing faith in her father.

I want to acknowledge my agent, Matthew Carnicelli, the first "outsider" to show enthusiasm for the memoir; John Paine, who labored so diligently to edit early versions; Debra Englander at Post Hill who never lost her passion for the story; Heather King, Allie Woodlee, and Madeline Sturgeon who edited the work into coherence; and Suzanne and Elliot Balaban at BMM Worldwide who used their gentle but firm hand to guide me into the public space.

I owe a special debt of gratitude to first readers who, to my astonishment, liked the work and urged me to continue to refine it: Lynn White, Anna Wells, Joni Clemons, Jim Clemons, Lorraine Egan, Bill Egan, David St. Geme, Thomas St. Geme, Deb Schrag, Christopher Slapak, Michael Robertson, Ralph Blair, Pam Peck, Ellen Nigrosh, Robin Weiss, Richard Ransohoff, Becky Ruthven, Jeff Jacobs, Steve Koppel, Ellen Ziffren, Aimee Bell, Emily Cunningham, and Frederick Ruf.

Finally, I want to thank Jane's colleagues and friends, those who loved her and helped her through her final year: Michael Robertson, Christopher Slapak, Deb Schrag, Chuck Stiles, Roz Segal, Ed

Benz, Peggy Vettese, David Nathan, Eric Winer, Susan Block, Rob Soiffer, Larry Shulman, David Harrington, Margaret Shipp, Jennifer Mack, Gregory Abel, Michael Hassett, Rinaa Punglia, Judy Garber, Val Marsoobian, Nicole Kovil, Stephanie Patel, Dora Toledo, Jennifer McKenna, Deb DiPrete, Susan Troyan, Paul Sax, Gary Gilliland, Mace Rothenberg, Tom Lee, Soheyla Gharib, Bob Mayer, Jim Griffin, Craig Bunnell, Rodolfo Silva, Cynthia and Grant Schaumburg, Nestor Real, Bonnie Lesser, and Wendy Gettleman.

ABOUT THE AUTHOR

Barrett Rollins is an oncologist and cancer researcher who has published over one hundred scholarly articles, chapters, and books. He is the Linde Family Professor of Medicine at Harvard Medical School and was, for sixteen years, chief scientific officer at Dana-Farber Cancer Institute. Born and raised in Cleveland, he graduated from Amherst College—which also gave him an honorary Doctor of Science—and received his M.D. and Ph.D. from Case Western Reserve University where he was honored with its Distinguished Alumni Award. He is a long-time trustee of the Interlochen Center for the Arts and lives in Boston with his wife Lynn and their dogs, Skyler and Zeke.